CAMBRIDGE STUDIES IN
ANGLO-SAXON ENGLAND

7

ANGLO-SAXON MEDICINE

CAMBRIDGE STUDIES IN
ANGLO-SAXON ENGLAND

EDITORS

SIMON KEYNES

MICHAEL LAPIDGE

Editors' preface

Cambridge Studies in Anglo-Saxon England is a series of scholarly texts and monographs intended to advance our knowledge of all aspects of the field of Anglo-Saxon studies. The scope of the series, like that of *Anglo-Saxon England*, its periodical counterpart, embraces original scholarship in various disciplines: literary, historical, archaeological, philological, art historical, palaeographical, architectural, liturgical and numismatic. It is the intention of the editors to encourage the publication of original scholarship which advances our understanding of the field through interdisciplinary approaches.

Volumes published

ANGLO-SAXON MEDICINE

M. L. CAMERON
Professor (Retired) of Biology,
Dalhousie University

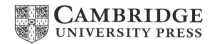

CAMBRIDGE
UNIVERSITY PRESS

Published by the Press Syndicate of the University of Cambridge
The Pitt Building, Trumpington Street, Cambridge CB2 1RP
40 West 20th Street, New York, NY 10011-4211, USA
10 Stamford Road, Oakleigh, Melbourne 3166, Australia

First published 1993

Printed in Great Britain at the University Press, Cambridge

A catalogue record for this book is available from the British Library

Library of Congress cataloguing in publication data
Cameron, M. L. (Malcolm Laurence), 1918–
Anglo-saxon medicine / M. L. Cameron.
p.   cm. (Cambridge Studies in Anglo-Saxon England)
Includes bibliographical references and index.
ISBN 0 521 40521 1 (hardback)
1. Anglo-Saxons – Medicine.   I. Title.
R141.C35   1993
615.8'99'09 – dc20   92–29974 CIP

ISBN 0 521 40521 1 hardback

For my Mother,
for her 100th birthday

Contents

Contents

Preface

The present book is an attempt to explain the rational basis of Anglo-Saxon medicine in the light of modern physiology and pharmacology. I should explain at the outset why I have undertaken this approach, and I think I should offer some explanation of my educational background. My formal education and training have been in biology, especially in limnology (the dynamics of the evolution of fresh-water lakes) and in invertebrate physiology. I have never had a lesson in Old English or in the history of Anglo-Saxon England; all I know about these subjects I have acquired through my interest in medieval medicine. I should perhaps add that I spent my childhood on a farm where the children were expected to be able to identify all the animals and plants around them. We lived with a grandmother whose memory went back to the way of life of Scottish Highland crofters transplanted to the New World. It was a way of life, I have come to realize, not very different from that of the Anglo-Saxons.

As a consequence, I entered on the study of Anglo-Saxon medicine, being deficient in much of importance in Anglo-Saxon language, literature and history, but at the same time having a background rich in ancient folk-customs and mores experienced at first hand, and an understanding of the scientific bases of disease, therapeutics and pharmacology. Because I think that this background has given me a peculiar outlook on the subject of Anglo-Saxon medicine, I have dared to write this book. I am very much aware that my deficiencies in formal training in Anglo-Saxon studies expose me to the expression of opinions and conclusions which would not be committed by one with better training, yet I hope that these errors will inspire others, more capable than I am, to correct them and by so doing advance our knowledge of a fascinating and important part of the English heritage.

Acknowledgements

It is always a pleasure to acknowledge help which one has received, and in the making of this book I have many people and institutions to thank. If there are ones I have inadvertently omitted, I beg their pardon while I acknowledge their aid.

First of all, I thank Dalhousie University and the Killam Trust for their grants in aid of research, which enabled me to spend sabbatical leaves in the Cambridge University Library, the libraries of Trinity College and Peterhouse, Cambridge, and the British Library. To these libraries and their librarians I give my warm thanks for their unfailing courtesy and help over many years. More recently, the generous grants for travel and research given by the Hannah Institute for the History of Medicine have enabled me to continue my work in these libraries.

I have also to thank very many people who have been generous in helping me in many ways. First of all I must express my gratitude to a former teacher, J. A. Livingstone, who long ago taught me how to study properly, a lesson without which I should never have done anything useful. Colleagues who have given of their time and knowledge freely are: Professors Linda Voigts, Audrey Meaney and Maria (Maila) D'Aronco, and the members of the Dictionary of Old English at the University of Toronto (but especially Dr Pauline Thompson).

I should never have become interested in Anglo-Saxon studies were it not for Professor Peter A. M. Clemoes, who, when we were students together, introduced me, quite unwittingly on his part, to their fascination. Later it was Professor Clemoes who also introduced me to the intricacies of writing for publication in the humanities (quite a revelation for one who had previously been trained only in the natural sciences). It was he also who introduced me to Professor Michael Lapidge, than whom there can be no more understanding and helpful editor. I wish also to thank Sarah Stanton and Jenny Potts for their kind help in the production of the book.

Above all I thank my wife, who has been my best critic at all times.

Abbreviations

ASE	*Anglo-Saxon England*
ASPR	*Anglo-Saxon Poetic Records*, ed. G. P. Krapp and E. V. K. Dobbie, 6 vols. (New York, 1931–42)
BL	British Library
CCSL	Corpus Christianorum, Series Latina (Turnhout)
CH	*Curae herbarum*
CUL	Cambridge University Library
EETS os	Early English Text Society, Original Series
EHF	*Ex herbis femininis*
HE	Bede's *Ecclesiastical History of the English People*, ed. Colgrave and Mynors
MDQ	*Medicina de quadrupedibus*
MGH	Monumenta Germaniae Historica
PL	Patrologia Latina, ed. J. P. Migne, 221 vols. (Paris, 1844–64)
Pliny, *HN*	*Pliny, Natural History*, ed. Jones
QM	*Quaestiones medicinales*

1

Introduction

The world's oldest medical text is a clay tablet from Ur inscribed some 4,000 years ago. The oldest surviving Egyptian medical text is the Kahun papyrus, which was written about 150 years later. The oldest surviving Greek texts are copies of the writings of Hippocrates of Cos, who flourished about 400 BC and was contemporary with Socrates and Plato. Copies of later Greek and Latin medical texts are plentiful, including the three volumes of the works of Celsus in Latin and the twenty volumes of the works of Galen in Greek. The result is that we have a very fair sample of the medical lore of the Mediterranean world from a very early date. But before 1100 north of the Alps only one culture has left us anything of its own; uniquely among Northern Europeans the Anglo-Saxons appear from early times to have written medical texts in their own language as well as in Latin, and enough of these have survived from the tenth century and later to give us a good picture of what medicine was like in a northern country in medieval times.

Their Latin texts are almost entirely copies, or direct derivatives, of Latin ones originating in the Mediterranean regions of Europe, Asia and North Africa, and so are of greatest interest in showing the contacts between the Anglo-Saxons and the cultures of those regions. On the other hand, the surviving Old English texts are unique among European medical records. Whereas other surviving medical writings up to the end of the eleventh century were composed in Greek (in Eastern Europe) or in Latin (in the West and in North Africa), only in England was there an extensive medical literature in a vernacular language. This Old English material contains both translations from the Latin and, more importantly, original compilations containing much native medicine. As a consequence, we are in the fortunate position today of being able to assess the medical practices

1

and beliefs of a Northern European people and to compare them with the more classically derived Latin and Greek material. Although the oldest surviving medical documents in Old English are not earlier than the late ninth century, there is evidence that older ones have been lost and that the practice of writing medical works in the vernacular was practised by the Anglo-Saxons from an earlier time.

Considering how great has been the loss of manuscripts since Anglo-Saxon times, the thousand or more manuscript pages on medical themes in Old English which remain, making up as they do an appreciable part of the corpus of surviving writings in Old English, attest to the considerable importance of medicine to the Anglo-Saxons. If to these remains in Old English we add the Latin texts compiled by Anglo-Saxons, we have a unique opportunity to evaluate their medical practices. And because a very large amount of medical material survives in manuscripts of Greek, Roman, North African and Byzantine origins, we also have the opportunity to compare Anglo-Saxon medicine with that of these Mediterranean cultures and to assess their influence on it.

There has been an unfortunate and widely held belief that all ancient medicine, with the exception of that of the Hippocratic school, of Galen and of some early Byzantine physicians, was filled with superstitious and magical practices and with generally worthless remedies, practices and theories, until the awakening of interest in Greek and Roman medicine at the school of Salerno in the tenth and eleventh centuries. It was this belief which prompted Charles Singer to write in 1952: 'Surveying the mass of folly and credulity that makes up A.S. leechdoms, it may be asked, "Is there any rational element here? Is the material based on anything that we may describe as experience?" The answer must be "Very little."'[1] But John Riddle has recently criticized judiciously this way of thinking: 'For too long we have believed that the past was filled more with superstition and stupidities than with experienced judgements about medicine.'[2]

Singer had based his opinion of Anglo-Saxon medicine largely on a close study of the thoroughly unscholarly *Lacnunga*, and was clearly prejudiced in his judgement. But other commentators on the culture and literature of the Anglo-Saxons, undoubtedly misled by comments such as those of Singer, have been no kinder. One of these gave a single short paragraph to their medicine, which began: 'Several other manuscripts containing

[1] In Grattan and Singer, *Anglo-Saxon Magic*, p. 92.

[2] J. R. Riddle, 'Ancient and Medieval Chemotherapy for Cancer', *Isis* 76 (1985), 319–30.

pseudo-scientific material survive from the later part of the Anglo-Saxon period.' and ended with a quotation from Singer: 'So far from containing any rational element which might mark the beginnings of scientific advance, "it is the last stage of a process that has left no legitimate successor, a final pathological disintegration of the great system of Greek medical thought".'3 Another commentator on the history of Old English literature dismissed the medical texts thus: 'Medical theory and practice, from the evidence of this text [Bald's *Leechbook*] and of others, especially the *Lacnunga*, was primarily a curious mixture of degenerated knowledge of Greek medicine, Teutonic pagan charms, and Latin Christian overlay that merits more the name of magic than of medicine.'4

As long ago as 1904 Joseph Payne had condemned this attitude:

Too often, those few persons who have interested themselves in these monuments of ancient science have treated them in one of two ways. Either they have picked out something especially unlike the ways of modern thought, and held it up to scorn as showing the folly of our ancestors, or else in kinder mood they have condescended to be amused, and calling anything old and unfamiliar 'quaint', dismissed it with a smile.

He added:

The only way to understand these old writers is to try to put ourselves as far as possible in their place, and conceive how nature and science presented themselves in the eyes of the early teacher and learner in the tenth and eleventh centuries . . . That they tried to understand them at all is a proof of their wisdom, not of their folly.5

It is obvious that we have here two completely opposed views of the content and quality of Anglo-Saxon medicine, Singer and his followers on the one hand finding in it only masses of superstition and folly, and Payne and Riddle on the other seeing it worthy of sympathetic appraisal. I shall try to follow Payne's advice to put myself and the reader of this book in a position to appreciate the medical views of the Anglo-Saxons. To do this,

---

3 P. H. Blair, *An Introduction to Anglo-Saxon England* (Cambridge, 1956), pp. 360–1. (Singer's quotation was removed from the second edition of 1977.)

4 S. B. Greenfield, *A Critical History of Old English Literature* (New York, 1965), pp. 61–2. These sentiments were removed from Greenfield and D. G. Calder, *A New Critical History of Old English Literature* (New York, 1986); see pp. 116–17 for a more sympathetic view of Anglo-Saxon medicine.

5 J. F. Payne, *English Medicine*, pp. 38–9.

we must examine the whole corpus of their medicine to determine, as far as we may, its sources in classical and in native Teutonic medical practices, and to assess its quality as useful medicine in comparison with the practices of the Greeks and Romans and their North African and Byzantine followers. By so doing, we should arrive at an assessment of its value as medicine in the context of its time and place, and thus be able to decide between the positions of Singer and Payne, always keeping in mind Payne's advice to put ourselves as far as possible in the Anglo-Saxons' place, and to arrive at our assessments through the medical and physiological background of their time, not of ours.

In contrast to the neglect of rational medical components of Anglo-Saxon medicine, its magical component has received much attention, and important work has been done on it, so that a one-sided picture has emerged. Recently, in the spirit of Payne's advice, students of medieval medicine have begun to examine its rational components and to study the medical value of their remedies. Because this approach is recent and only a handful of workers are applying it, it is inevitable that this present study must be in many ways tentative and opinionated. I shall feel amply rewarded if what I present here convinces others that Anglo-Saxon medicine deserves sympathetic consideration.

Wishing that this monograph may be of some use to scholars in various fields with a minimum of effort on their part, I have quoted extensively from pertinent Old English, Greek and Latin materials, and have put in the text my own translations of these quotations, relegating the originals to footnotes or appendices. By this arrangement I have tried to make it possible for a reader not acquainted with the languages involved, or not having the original texts to hand, to read without interruption, and for one who wishes to have the originals to be able to refer to them easily, rather than having to go to editions, some of which are not easily come by, or to materials which exist only in manuscript. I hope that it will persuade some of them to undertake further unprejudiced studies in this fascinating field.

2

Conditions for health and disease

Before examining the medical records and their sources, we will find it helpful first to consider what we know (and may infer) about the conditions under which the Anglo-Saxons lived their daily lives, what were some of the ailments with which they were afflicted and how they treated them. The contents of grave sites reveal a fairly short life expectancy, a high infant mortality, women dying young, particularly in child-birth, and a fairly high incidence of bone and joint diseases, such as rheumatism, arthritis and rickets.[1] The Anglo-Saxon population cannot have been particularly healthy. The conditions of life and diet help to establish a background for many of their illnesses.

Housing was relatively primitive, especially for a northern climate, and there is no doubt that we should have found their dwellings most uncomfortable. Archaeological evidence shows that most persons lived in small, damp, dark hovels, probably of one room, heated by a fire on a central hearth, with an opening in the roof through which smoke was supposed to escape.[2] That the dwellings of the most affluent could not have been much more comfortable we learn from Bede's account of the council at the court of King Edwin of Northumbria in 627, concerning the adoption of the Christian faith, during which a councillor gave a beautiful description of the brevity of human life. He said:

The present life of man on earth, O king, in comparison with the time which is unknown to us, seems to me as when you sit at dinner with your commanders and ministers in winter time, with a fire burning on the hearth in the midst in a good warm dining-hall while everywhere outside the rains or snows of winter are raging,

[1] V. Bullough and C. Campbell, 'Female Longevity and Diet in the Middle Ages', *Speculum* 55 (1980), 317–25.
[2] P. V. Addyman, 'The Anglo-Saxon House: a New Review', *ASE* 1 (1972), 273–307.

a sparrow should come in and fly quickly through the room, who when it has entered by one door soon leaves by another. While it is inside it is not touched by the winter storm, but after a short time of calm gone in a moment, at once it slips from your sight returning from winter to winter.[3]

What interests us here is not the councillor's striking comparison, but the fact that even a king's hall in a mid-winter storm had its doors so open that birds could fly through; it is not hard to imagine the draughts which must also have blown from open door to open door through the 'good warm dining-hall'. The peasant's cottage was probably no more exposed to the weather. When people lived under such conditions, it is not to be wondered at that their resistance to disease must have been impaired and that joint ailments, for example, must have been common.

The diet of a people plays a large part in the condition of its health. We do not have much information about the daily diet of the Anglo-Saxons, but a little can be gleaned here and there. We can infer from the foods mentioned in the medical records which ones were likely to be available. For instance, the most frequently mentioned grains are wheat and barley; rye is mentioned occasionally and oats only a couple of times and only in Bald's *Leechbook*. Bread is mentioned a number of times, sometimes without qualification, sometimes as leavened bread and occasionally as bread prepared from fine white wheaten flour. Legumes are mentioned often, most frequently beans (*Vicia faba*), known in England since the Iron Age, and peas (*Pisum sativum*) brought to Britain by the Romans. Lentils (*Lens esculentum*) are mentioned only twice and were probably not much grown in England. Legumes would provide important nourishment in a simple diet, particularly if combined with cereals, when their essential amino acid contents would complement those of the grains to provide a protein diet almost equivalent in food value to eggs, meat or milk. This combination of legumes and grains is an almost universal food practice, as

[3] *HE* II.15; ed. Colgrave and Mynors, pp. 182–5: 'Talis mihi uidetur, rex, uita hominum praesens in terris, ad conparationem eius, quod nobis incertum est, temporis, quale cum te residente ad caenam cum ducibus ac ministris tuis tempore brumali, accenso quidem foco in medio, et calido effecto caenaculo, furentibus autem foris per omnia turbinibus hiemalium pluuiarum uel niuium, adueniens unus passerum domum citissime peruolauerit; qui cum per unum ostium ingrediens, mox per aliud exierit. Ipso quidem tempore, quo intus est, hiemis tempestate non tangitur, sed tamen paruissimo spatio serenitatis ad momentum excurso, mox de hieme in hiemem regrediens, tuis oculis elabitur.'

we find it in the baked beans and corn bread of North America and the beans on toast of the English breakfast. It is unlikely that anyone in Anglo-Saxon England who got enough to eat should have suffered from serious protein deficiencies.

An informative source for dietary habits is found in the *Colloquy* of Ælfric, where in part of the conversation between the master and a student taking the role of a boy in a monastery we get an idea of what a lad in such a situation might expect to eat:

What do you eat in a day? – Until now I eat meat, because I am a boy living under discipline. – What more do you eat? – I eat vegetables and eggs, fish and cheese, butter and beans and everything clean – And what do you drink? – Ale, if I have it, or water if I do not have ale. – Do you not drink wine? – I am not so rich that I can buy wine for myself.[4]

For those who could get it, this would have been a well-balanced diet.

Elsewhere in the *Colloquy* we learn that there were shepherds and goat-herds. From the shepherd we learn the chief source of butter and cheese: 'Early in the morning I drive my sheep to pasture and stand over them in heat and cold with my dogs so that wolves may not devour them, and I lead them back to the folds and I milk them twice a day and move their folds and besides that I make cheese and butter.'[5] From this it appears that butter and cheese were commonly made from sheep's milk, which helps to explain specific references to 'cow's butter' in some of the medical recipes.

According to the *Colloquy* the fisherman caught eels, pike, minnows, burbots, trout and lampreys and whatever swam in the water, and sometimes ventured to sea, where he caught herrings, salmon, dolphins, sturgeon, oysters, crabs, mussels, winkles, cockles, plaice and flounder, lobsters and the like.[6] The hunter took wild deer and pigs and hares, which

---

[4] *Ælfric's Colloquy*, ed. Garmonsway, pp. 45–7: 'Quid manducas in die? – Adhuc carnibus uescor, quia puer sum sub uirga degens. – Quid plus manducas? – Holera et oua, pisces et caseum, butirum et fabas et omnia munda manduco . . . – Et quid bibis? – Ceruisam, si habeo, uel aquam si non habeo ceruisam. – Nonne bibis uinum? – Non sum tam diues ut possim emere mihi uinum.'

[5] *Ibid.*, p. 22: 'In primo mane meno oues meas ad pascua, et sto super eas in estu et frigore cum canibus, ne lupi deuorent eas, et reduco eas ad caulas, et mulgeo eas bis in die, et caulas earum moueo, insuper et caseum et butirum facio.'

[6] *Ibid.*, pp. 27–9: 'Anguillas et lucios, menas et capitones, tructas et murenas et qualescumque in amne natant . . . Alleces et isicios, delfinos et sturias, ostreas et cancros, musculas, torniculi, neptigalli, platesia et platissa et polipodes et similia.'

were for the use of his lord's table, the fowler caught birds but the kinds were not named.[7]

The same impression of a plentiful supply of corn for workers on an estate, but less indication of a good supply of meats, at least for the lower servants, is given by an estate memorandum of the tenth or eleventh century. During good years such servants may have fed adequately, although they were probably getting somewhat less meat than needed for a balanced diet.[8]

The evidence of the Old English *Leechbooks* supports these extracts from the *Colloquy* and memorandum. Bacon is mentioned a few times, as are hares and deer. Hens, geese and their eggs are mentioned often, pigeons occasionally. Milk and butter are among the most common ingredients in medicines, cream is mentioned a few times, as are cheese and curds and whey. Ale seems to have been the commonest drink, followed by beer and wine. As far as I know, mead is mentioned only twice. Of green vegetables, cabbages, which would certainly include winter forms such as kale, and cresses (watercress, garden cress, winter cress) and lettuce are the most frequently mentioned. Onions, leeks, garlic and radish are mentioned frequently, turnip and beet less often. It is difficult to distinguish in the texts between carrots and parsnips, but considered as a group they are frequently mentioned. Cucumbers are mentioned a few times; it is doubtful that they were commonly grown. Apples are the most commonly mentioned tree fruit; plums, cherries, sloes, rowan berries much less often. It is not clear whether the pear is mentioned more than once (one or two other possible references depend on textual emendation). Strawberries, raspberries and blackberries are frequently mentioned. The very frequent references to wine imply that grapes were grown in England or that there was a large import from the Continent. Of condiments and culinary herbs mentioned the most commonly available would have been mustards, coriander, cumin, dill, fennel, anise, parsley, lovage, chervil, celery (smallage), savory, various mints, sage, thyme, rosemary and tansy, all of which were native to England or could be grown there without difficulty. Honey, oil (kinds rarely specified) and vinegar are frequently mentioned.

It is doubtful, however, that most people did get enough of the right

[7] *Ibid.*, pp. 23–5 and 30–2.

[8] *Anglo-Saxon Prose*, ed. M. Swanton (Totowa, NJ, 1975), pp. 21–5. This is a translation of memoranda ed. F. Liebermann, *Die Gesetze der Angelsachsen*, 3 vols. (Halle, 1903–16) I, 446–53.

foods, particularly in winter and in years of poor crops, so that ailments resulting from deficiencies in diet must have been common, even apart from those resulting from an actual shortage of food. On a diet poor in red meats, it would have been difficult to get a sufficient supply of some vitamins and in winter, unless one could depend on having such green things as cabbages and kale, Vitamin C must have been in short supply. There is evidence that deficiencies of Vitamins A and C and of niacin were common enough to lead to the skin and eye problems grouped under the name *þeor*.[9] All these dietary deficiencies may have been usually subclinical in themselves, but would certainly lower resistance to disease.

Together with poor housing and dietary deficiencies, working conditions did much to contribute to many ailments. Again from the *Colloquy* we learn of the ploughman's daily routine:

Oh, my lord, I work too hard. I go out at break of day driving the oxen to the field and I yoke them to the plough. There is no winter so harsh that I dare to lurk at home for fear of my lord, but with yoked oxen and share and coulter fastened to the plough, every day I must plough an acre or more. – Have you any companion? – I have a boy driving the oxen with a goad, who now too is just as hoarse from cold and shouting. – What more do you do in a day? – To be sure I do more yet. I must fill the oxen's manger with hay and water them and carry out their manure.[10]

Similarly, the shepherd drove out his sheep at dawn to pasture and stood over them in heat and cold with his dogs, the ox-herd took the ploughman's team to pasture and watched over the oxen all night and brought them back to the ploughman at dawn fed and watered. Inadequately clothed and poorly fed as they must often have been, these workers were in no condition to withstand any onset of illness or disease and must have lived short and sorry lives.

What were some of the diseases to which they fell prey and how did they treat them? Here the Old English medical texts are invaluable. As we shall

---

[9] M. L. Cameron, 'On *þeor* and *þeoradl*', *Anglia* 106 (1988), 124–9.

[10] *Ælfric's Colloquy*, ed. Garmonsway, pp. 20–1: 'O, mi domine, nimium laboro. Exeo diluculo minando boues ad campum, et iungo eos ad aratrum; non est tam aspera hiems ut audeam latere domi pro timore domini mei, sed iunctis bobus, et confirmato uomere et cultro aratro, omni die debeo arare integrum agrum aut plus. – Habes aliquem socium? – Habeo quendam puerum minantem boues cum stimulo, qui etiam modo raucus est pre frigore et clamatione. – Quid amplius facis in die? – Certe adhuc plus facio. Debeo implere presepia boum feno, et adaquare eos, et fimum eorum portare foras.'

see in chs. 12 and 13, medieval people had some idea of infective disease; the frequent references to *flying venom*, to *elfshot* and to the *loathly one that roams through the land* can best be explained as showing an understanding of communicable diseases. The many references to dysentery imply that it was common enough to call for the reporting of many treatments, including magic ones. *Entamoeba histolytica* had ideal conditions for transmission in a society which did not know of its existence and which was not noted for its attention to personal and community hygiene. For similar reasons, infection by sheep liver fluke, *Fasciola hepatica*, must have occurred often in a society where sheep were kept in every community and watercress was gathered from streams adjoining sheep pastures. In the chapters on disease of the liver in Bald's *Leechbook*, there is evidence that invasions of the liver by both *Entamoeba* and *Fasciola* were known. Cirrhosis, vomiting, diarrhoea and abdominal rigidity, described in II.xxi, are consistent with liver fluke infection, just as chills, vomiting, enlargement and abscess of the liver, soreness of the abdomen, described in II.xvii, are consistent with infection by *Entamoeba histolytica*.[11] There is naturally no hint in these chapters or elsewhere that these liver conditions were associated with parasitic invasions.

A frequently mentioned disease was *lencten adl* ('spring ailment' or 'spring fever'). It seems clear that this name most commonly described an endemic form of tertian malaria, one in which the parasite remained dormant during much of the year, becoming active in spring about the same time as the adult forms of the mosquito vector emerged. The last case to be studied clinically was that of a young military recruit from the Romney district in 1911, the disease dying out as marshes and fens were drained, removing the mosquito's habitats. In the fen district of East Anglia in the eighteenth and early nineteenth centuries it was not unknown for a man to have had more than three wives, one child by each, the woman dying in childbearing not only because of the malaria but also because of the severe anaemia brought on by a combination of deficiency of iron in the diet, loss of iron from the malarial infection and removal of iron from the mother's body by the foetus.[12]

Although there are numerous remedies for *dweorg* ('fever'), only in Bald's *Leechbook* are there chapters on *lencten adl* and other forms of malaria. Very little could be done for those suffering from malarial fevers and the

[11] *Leechdoms*, ed. Cockayne II, 204–6 and 196–8.
[12] See MacArthur, 'English Malaria', *passim*.

remedies suggested were mostly herbal preparations to be drunk either during the attack or before it; most of these potions contained betony (*Stachys betonica*), whatever other herbs were in them. These potions must have been ineffective, because complicated magical remedies were also resorted to, and were most likely equally ineffective.

It is clear from the space given in the *Leechbooks* to ailments of the eyes that these were common and serious. It is difficult today to appreciate the problems of defective vision in a time before the invention of spectacles, but there were also those diseases of the eyes caused by unsanitary conditions leading to infections. Although these conditions could not have been as severe in England as in the drier and dustier south, the smoky atmosphere in dwellings having no chimneys must have led to much irritation of the eyes and increased the chances of infection. There is ample evidence from the large number of remedies for such ailments in the *Leechbooks* and *Lacnunga* that they were well known. In ch. 10, where somewhat less than half of the chapter on eye ailments is given from Bald's *Leechbook*, all the nineteen remedies quoted are for *eagena miste* ('mistiness of the eyes', 'dimness of vision'), which might describe astigmatism and poor accommodation, but more frequently referred to inflammations of the eye, scarring of the cornea and similar accidents resulting from infections and injuries of the eye. Later remedies in the same chapter are for *eagece* ('pain in the eyes'), *flie* (albugo, that is, white spot on the cornea and also cataract), watering of the eyes, styes, *æsmæl* (probably 'shrinkage of the eyeball'), *worms* in the eyes, *þeoradl on eagum* ('xerophthalmia', 'trachoma') and inflamed and infected eyelids.

For most of these troubles not much could be done; we shall see that some infections were treated with antibiotic preparations which may have been of some help. For the presbyopia of advancing age, this was the best that was offered: 'An old person's eyes are not sharpsighted. Then he is to arouse his eyes with rubbings, with walkings, with ridings, either when he is carried or taken in a wagon, and they are to use foods sparingly and timid(?) ones and comb their heads and drink wormwood before taking food.'[13] This advice came from Oribasius (Greek, fourth century AD), who got it from earlier writers; almost the same words were written by Celsus

---

[13] *Leechdoms*, ed. Cockayne II, 30–2: 'Ealdes mannes eagan beoþ unscearpsyno; þonne sceal he þa eagan weccan mid gnidingum, mid gongum, mid radum, oþþe mid þy þe hine mon bere oþþe on wæne ferige; 7 hy sculan nyttian lytlum 7 forhtlicum metum 7 hiora heafod cemban 7 wermod drincan ær þon þe hie mete þicgean.'

(Roman, first century AD). The fact remains that the active working period of anyone who depended on sharp vision was much shorter than it is today. The *Petrocellus* has a treatment, translated (incorrectly) into the late Old English *Peri Didaxeon*, which, although it may not be in the direct line of Anglo-Saxon medicine, is worth quoting: 'Nyctalopia of the eyes, that is one who cannot see after sunset until sunrise: Roasted buck liver, from which a liquid flows out when it is roasted; anoint the eyes with it and give the liver itself to be eaten.'[14] There is no doubt that the eating of liver would supply Vitamin A, a deficiency of which is the chief cause of night blindness. How such a remedy was discovered is a fascinating question. But the writer followed this sensible treatment with the following one: 'and fresh ass's dung strained through a linen cloth, anoint with it.'[15]

We must bear in mind that there was no adequate anaesthesia until the nineteenth century and there is evidence that Anglo-Saxons were aware only of the anodyne properties of some herbs such as mandrake, henbane and poppy. In consequence, ailments such as toothache had to be endured, and an examination of remedies for it shows how inadequate they were. Typical are a couple from *Leechbook III*: 'For toothache chew pepper with the tooth; it will soon be well. Again: cook henbane roots in strong vinegar or in wine, set on the sore tooth and from time to time chew with the sore tooth; it will be well.'[16] But with no way to treat an abscessed tooth or to extract it, these palliative measures gave only temporary relief. In medieval medicine there was a continuing belief that tooth decay was caused by worms and medicines were prescribed for getting rid of them: 'For tooth worms, take oak meal and henbane seed and wax, equal amounts of all, mix together, make into a wax candle and burn it, let it smoke into the mouth, put a black sheet under, then the worms will fall on it.'[17]

There were many treatments for ailments of the ears; as Bald's *Leechbook* put it: 'Medicines for all pains and ache of the ears and for deafness of the

[14] M. Löweneck, 'Peri Didaxeon', pp. 1–57, at 14: 'Nuctolopas oculorum, id est que post solis occasum usque ad ortum uidere prohibet: Epar hircini assum, ex ipso enim dum assatur humor fluit; ex inde oculos unguis et ipsum epar das ad manducandum.'

[15] *Ibid.*: 'et asininum fimum recentem per linteum colatum, ex inde inunguis'.

[16] *Leechdoms*, ed. Cockayne II, 310: 'Wiþ toþece ceow pipor gelome mid þam toþum, him biþ sona sel. Eft: seoð beolenan moran on strangum ecede oþþe on wine, sete on þone saran toþ 7 hwilum ceowe mid þy saran toþe; he bit hal.'

[17] *Ibid.*, p. 50: 'Wiþ toð wyrmum, genim ac mela 7 beolonan sæd 7 weax, ealra emfela, meng tosomne, wyrc to weax candelle 7 bærn, læt reocan on þone muð, do blæc hrægl under, þonne feallaþ þa wyrmas on.'

ears and if worms or earwigs are in the ears and if there is a dinning in the ears and ear salves.'[18] Sore ears were treated with warm oil in which various herbs were infused or with lukewarm henbane juice dripped into the ear. Bile of various animals was used for deafness, and for dinning in the ears a plug of wool dipped in oil was put in the ear overnight. Many of these medicines came from Latin and Greek sources; one which was widespread until at least the fifteenth century was the following for earache: 'Take a rod of green ash, lay it in the fire, then take the juice which comes out of it, put on wool, wring into the ear and with the same wool stop up the ear.'[19] Some of these remedies may have given relief if only because they were applied warm.

Rheumatoid arthritis and rickets, as indicated by grave remains, were not uncommon and, indeed, there are many recipes for treating pains in the limbs and joints. Again, treatment could only be palliative: 'If a knee is sore, pound henbane and hemlock, foment with it and lay it on.'[20] 'For pain in the thigh [presumably sciatica]: smoke the thighs thoroughly with fern.'[21] Broken limbs were bathed and anointed with salves; splints are mentioned only twice: 'For a broken limb, put this salve on the broken limb and cover it with elm bark, apply a splint, afterwards constantly renew until it is healed. Peel elm bark and boil thoroughly, then remove the bark, take linseed, grind [into a] poultice with the "drink" of the elm; it will be a good salve for a broken limb.'[22] 'For many a person his feet contract to his hams. Prepare a bath, add bitter vetch and cress and the small nettle and sweet flag, put into a trough hot stones well heated, bathe the hams with the stone bath; when they are sweating then let him stretch the bones as well as he can, put on a splint and it is better the oftener one bathes with it.'[23] Presumably this treatment was for a fractured thigh. All

[18] *Ibid.*, pp. 38–40: 'Læcedomas wið eallum earena sare 7 ece 7 wið earena adeafunge 7 gif wyrmas on earan synd oþþe earwicga 7 gif earan dynien 7 earsealfa.'

[19] *Ibid.*, p. 42: 'Genim grenne æscenne stæf, lege on fyr, genim þonne þæt seaw þe him of gæþ, do on þa ilcan wulle, wring on eare 7 mid þære ilcan wulle forstoppa þæt eare.'

[20] *Ibid.*, p. 340: 'Gif cneow sar sie cnua beolenan 7 hemlic, beþe mid 7 lege on.'

[21] *Ibid.*, p. 64: 'Wiþ þeoh ece: smice mid fearne swiþe þa þeoh.'

[22] *Ibid.*, p. 66: 'Wið foredum lime, lege þas sealfe on þæt forode lim 7 forlege mid elmrinde, do spilc to, eft simle niwa oþþæt gehalgod sie. Gerendra elmrinde 7 awyl swiðe, do þonne of þa rinde, genim linsæd, gegrind briwe wið þam elmes drænce; þæt bið god sealf foredum lime.'

[23] *Ibid.*, p. 68: 'Monegum men gescrincað his fet to his homme. Wyrc baþo, do earban to 7 cersan 7 smale netelan 7 beowyrt, do on troh hate stanas wel gehæette, gebeþe þa hamma

in all, treatment of broken bones did not do much to assure a sound limb after healing.

Another ailment for which not much could be done was paralysis, but various heroic measures were prescribed. One from *Leechbook III* is so elaborate it deserves quotation:

Take bramble bark and elm bark, ash bark, sloethorn bark, appletree bark, ivy bark (all these from the lower part) and cucumber, birthwort, polypody, elecampane, woody nightshade, betony, horehound, radish, agrimony; shred the herbs into a kettle and boil thoroughly; when it is thoroughly boiled take off the fire and set down and make a seat for the patient over the kettle and cover the patient up so that the steam cannot get out anywhere, except that the patient may be able to breathe. Foment him with this fomentation as long as he can endure it.[24]

Other treatments recommended were vomiting and bloodletting either by venesection or by cupping. None of these would have done anything useful for the sufferer.

Jaundice, *geolwan adl*, was usually treated with herbal potions, some-times with very complex remedies. However, there is in bk I of Bald's *Leechbook* a chapter on jaundice which gives more extensive treatment and is interesting also because it contains diagnostic symptoms:

From bile disease, that is from the yellow one, comes great misery. It is the most powerful of all diseases; then an excess of humour grows internally. These are the symptoms: that his body all becomes bitter and turns yellow like good silk and under his tongue strongly black and bad veins and his urine is yellow. Let him blood from the lung vein, give him often a stirring potion, stone baths frequently. Prepare for him then a calming drink of dock in wine and water, and every morning in the bath let him drink a mulled [sweetened] drink; it will alleviate the bitterness of the bile.[25]

    mid þam stanbaðe; þonne hie sien geswate þonne recce he þa ban swa he swiþost mæge, do spelc to 7 betere was mon oftor mid þy beþige.'

[24] *Ibid.*, p. 388: 'Genim bremblerinde 7 elmrinde, æscrinde, slahþornrinde, apuldorrinde, ifigrinde (ealle þas nioþowearde) 7 hwerhwettan, smeruwyrt, eoforfearn, elene ælfþone, betonice, marubie, redic, agrimonia; gescearfa þa wyrta on cetel 7 wyl swiðe; þonne hit sie swiþe gewylled do of þam fyre 7 sete 7 gewyrc þam men setl ofer þam citele 7 bewreow ðone man mid þæt se æþm ne mæge ut nahwær butan he mæge geeþian. Beþe hine mid þisse beþinge þa hwile þe he mæge aræfnan.'

[25] *Ibid.*, pp. 106–8: 'Of gealadle sio biþ of þære geolwan cymeþ great yfel. Sio biþ ealra adla ricust; þonne geweaxeð on innan ungemet wætan. Þis sint tacn: þæt him se lichoma eall abiterað 7 ageolwað swa god seoluc 7 him beoð under tungan tulge swearte ædra 7 yfele 7 him bið micge geolu. Læt him of lungen ædre blod, sele him oft styrgendne drenc,

A stone bath is recommended in another treatment also and a potion made up from dock in wine or water and sweetened. It is of interest that various kinds of dock (*Rumex* spp.) are still recommended in modern herbals as cholagogues for jaundice.

Chs. 46–50 of bk II of Bald's *Leechbook* deal with pains in the side and their treatment. This is a very interesting section of the *Leechbook* because in it an attempt is made to distinguish among various causes of pain in the side. Following a description of symptoms, by which pleurisy and perhaps pneumonia may be recognized, there is a section on prognosis:

If these symptoms continue for a long time, then the ailment is too dangerous and the patient cannot be cured. Nevertheless, ask the one who suffers this whether he ever was struck in the side or stabbed or whether some time before he had fallen or got a fracture. If it were that, then he will be easier to cure. If it comes from cold or from harmful internal humours it will be because of that harder to cure. Then if he had earlier suffered from pain in the liver or in the lungs and the pain in the side comes from that then is it very dangerous. If it had been earlier in the spleen then it is easier to cure. Then if he earlier had been wounded in the lung and the pain in the side comes from that, then that is very dangerous. If it had been earlier in the spleen then the pain comes in the left side, that also has serious danger; ask him whether his spleen is sore or whether he has a sore throat. Thus you may understand that pain in the side comes from harmful humours and is very dangerous . . . By these symptoms you may understand where the man is to be treated and where not.[26]

By using these methods of diagnosis the physician attempted to separate mechanical causes of pain in the side from pleurisy and pneumonia. His diagnostic details may have come from the Latin literature, but he was

stanbaðu gelome. Wyrc him ðonne stilne drenc of ompran on wine 7 on wætre, 7 on þam baðe gehwilce morgene drince mylsce drincan; sio gebet þa biternesse þæs geallan.'

[26] *Ibid.*, pp. 258–60: 'Gif þas tacn lange wuniað, þonne biþ seo adl to frecenlico 7 ne mæg him mon getilian. Ahsa hwæþre þone mannan þe þis þrowað hwæþer he æfre wære slegen on þa sidan oððe gestungen oþþe hwæþer he lenge ær afeolle oððe gebrocen wurde. Gif hit þæt wære þonne bið he þy eaðlæcna. Gif hit biþ of cyle cumen oþþe of yfelre inwætan hit bið þe uneaþlæcra. Gif he þonne biþ ær on þære lifre oþþe on þam lungenum gesargod 7 þanan cymeð sio sidwærc þonne biþ þæt swiðe frecne. Gif hit on þam milte biþ ær þonne biþ hit þy eaþlacre. Gif he þonne biþ ær on þære lungene gewundod 7 þanan cymð se sidwærc þonne biþ þæt swið frecne. Gif hit on þam milte bið ær þonne cymð þæt sar on þa winstran sidan, ge þa habbað hefige frecennesse; ahsa hine hwæþer him se milte sar sie oððe hwæþer him sweorcoþu sie. Swa þu meaht ongitan þæt þære sidan sar cymð of yfelre wætan 7 biþ swiðe frecne . . . Be þisum tacnum þu meaht hwær se man to lacnianne sie ongitan, hwær ne sie.'

perceptive enough to translate them for the advantage of English patients. It has been said repeatedly that such niceties of medical practice as diagnosis and prognosis were unknown to these Anglo-Saxon practitioners, but entries such as this one show that they were anxious and willing to use them when they could. The medieval physician was not indifferent to his patients' welfare; he simply had very little background on how living bodies behave and so his treatments were all too often of little or no use for the ailments he treated. For example, in the treatments which follow the diagnosis given here, cupping and venesection to remove harmful humours are among the important treatments he recommended.

Among the ailments discussed on a quire lost from Bald's *Leechbook* was *seo healfdeade adl* (the halfdead disease, hemiplegia). Cockayne found in another manuscript[27] an entry which gives a description of the symptoms leading to an identification of the disease and the methods of treatment:

The disease comes on the right side of the body or on the left; there the sinews are relaxed and have a slimy and thick humour, harmful, thick and plentiful. The humour must be removed with bloodlettings and potions and medicines. When the disease first comes on the patient, then open his mouth, look at his tongue; then it is whiter on the side on which the disease will be. Then treat him thus: Carry the patient into a very well enclosed and warm chamber, let him rest there very well sheltered and let warm coals be brought in frequently. Then unwrap him and look at his hands carefully and whichever one you find cold, at once bleed him on the cold vein.[28]

Following directions for several treatments, there is this paragraph, of which the first part has its source in the Latin *Liber tertius/Petrocellus*; the rest may be a statement by the compiler himself, an unusually rhetorical one in a book otherwise very impersonal:

Truly, the disease comes on a person after forty or fifty years; if he is of a cold temperament then it comes after forty, otherwise it comes after fifty years of his age. If it happens to a younger person then it is easier to cure and is not the same

---

[27] London, BL, Harley 55, 1r–3r. Cockayne identified the material on these folios as being a copy of some of the remedies lost from Bald's *Leechbook*.

[28] *Leechdoms*, ed. Cockayne II, 280: 'Seo adl cymð on þa swiðran healfe þæs lichoman oððe on þa wynstran; þær þa sina toslupað 7 beoð mid slipigre 7 þiccere wætan yfelre 7 yfelre þiccere 7 mycelre. Þa wætan man scæl mid blodlæsum 7 drencum 7 læcedomum on weg adon. Þonne seo adl cume ærest on ðone mannan þonne ontyne þu his muð, sceawa his tungan; þonne bið heo on þa healfe hwittre þe seo adl on beon wile. Lacna hine þonne þus: Gefere þæne mannan on swiðe fæstne cleofan 7 wearmne, gereste him swiðe wel hleowe

disease, although ignorant physicians think that it is the same halfdead disease. How can a similar disease befall one in youth on any limb as the halfdead disease does in old age? It is not the halfdead disease, but some other harmful humour has flooded the limb in which it settles, but it is easier to cure. But the real halfdead disease comes after fifty years.[29]

Whoever may have been responsible for this statement, it illustrates well the dangers of arguing from untested premises. According to humoral theory, phlegm (a slimy, thick humour) was apt to dominate in old age and was responsible for hemiplegia. The dominant humours in youth were blood and (in later years) bile, which were not responsible for hemiplegia. Therefore, even if a youth should show symptoms which were those of hemiplegia, he was deemed not to be suffering from hemiplegia but from some other humoral imbalance which had affected his limbs, and the proof that this was so was that the condition was more easily curable than the hemiplegia of old age. The humoral theory of illness put theories of disease and the practice of medicine into an intellectual prison from which escape was made only in the nineteenth century.

Insufficient iron in the diet is a situation frequently disregarded in assessing the health of a community. Shortage of dietary iron would have been particularly hard on women, whose requirement for iron in the diet during their child-bearing time of life is almost twice that of men, and during pregnancy even greater. It is likely that the average dietary supply of iron may have been minimal for males, so that for women it would have been chronically deficient.[30] In regions where malaria was endemic, this shortage of iron would have been even more serious, because of the excessive loss of red blood cells during malarial attacks and the consequent inability of the body to recover the iron from their haemoglobin.[31] The iron content of vegetables is low, and its availability usually less than 5 per cent of that present; only red meats have a high content in the haeme form

þær 7 wearme gleda bere man gelome inn. Onwreoh hine þonne 7 sceawa his handa georne 7 swa hwæþere swa ðe cealde finde læt him sona blod on þære cealdan ædre.'

[29] *Ibid.*, p. 284: 'Soðlice seo adl cymð on monnan æfter feowertigum oððe fiftigum wintra; gif he bið cealdre gecyndo þonne cymð æfter feowertigum, elcor cymð æfter fiftigum wintra his gærgetales. Gif hit gingran men gelimpe þonne bið þæt eaðlæcnere 7 ne bið seo ylce adl þeah þe ungleawe læcas wenan þæt þæt seo ylce healfdeade adl si. Hu gelic adl on man becume on geogoðe on sumum lime swa swa seo healfdeade adl on yldo deð? Ne bið hit seo healfdeade adl, ac hwilc æthwega yfel wæte bið gegoten on þæt lim þe hit on gesit, ac bið eaðlæcnere. Ac seo soðe healfdeade adl cymð æfter fiftigum wintra.'

[30] See above, p. 5, n. 1.   [31] MacArthur, 'English Malaria'.

which is readily assimilated. Vitamin C increases the assimilation of iron in non-haeme forms, but substances present in ·vegetables inhibit it. Moreover, as a result of malaria, iron is lost in excess from the body and what iron is present tends to be stored, rather than used for metabolic purposes. It is easy to see that a diet such as that of the Anglo-Saxons and the effects of endemic malaria would almost inevitably lead to iron deficiency. The worst aspect of this deficiency is that it leads to bodily weakness, greatly decreased ability to do a good day's work, difficulty in maintaining normal body temperature where the ambient temperature is low and, even more importantly, leads in growing children to central nervous problems and possible permanent damage to the brain with consequent lowering of intelligence. At any rate, a population deficient in iron is one which works and thinks below its inherent level of efficiency.[32]

The spleen is affected by the breakdown of red blood cells and consequent loss of iron from their haemoglobin and becomes enlarged in consequence. So common is this enlargement of the spleen in persons afflicted with malaria that physicians can estimate its incidence by simply palpating abdomens to determine the state of spleens. Bald's *Leechbook* has several chapters on ailments of the spleen. It is interesting that a remedy for enlarged spleen was a drink containing iron acetate prepared by plunging a red-hot poker or other iron rod into vinegar or wine.[33] How treatments such as this one and the eating of liver for night blindness were discovered are intriguing mysteries of ancient and folk medicines.

The examples of this chapter in no way cover all the ailments for which treatments are given in Anglo-Saxon treatises. They are intended only to illustrate the general picture of ailments and practice of medicine and to show the reader what one may expect when the Anglo-Saxon medical texts are examined. They also show that the methods of treatment for many of the ills from which Anglo-Saxons suffered were sometimes satisfactory but more often wholly useless or even pernicious. In this respect, Anglo-Saxon medicine differed not at all from medical practice in the rest of the Western world.

[32] N. S. Scrimshaw, 'Iron Deficiency', *Scientific American* 265.4 (October, 1991), 46–52.

[33] *Leechdoms*, ed. Cockayne II, 256: 'Læcedomas 7 swið drenc wiþ aswollenum milte: acele ðu wealhat isen þonne hit furthum sie of fiew atogen on wine oððe on ecede sele þæt drincan.' ('Remedies and a strong drink for swollen spleen: cool very hot iron when it is just taken from the fire in wine or in vinegar, give it to drink.')

3

Physician and patient

A weak man needs a physician.[1]

Before examining Anglo-Saxon medical literature in more detail, we should look at the physician and his patients. Unfortunately, we are told almost nothing about them. A little can be inferred from incidental references to physicians in various texts, but nowhere is one described nor his status made clear.

A few illustrations in illuminated manuscripts depict physicians at work. Most of them are shown in classical dress. But there are a couple showing physicians in native dress and untonsured, implying that they were not members of an ecclesiastical order.[2] If laymen were physicians, they must have been reasonably well educated, as surviving medical documents draw generously on Latin medical texts and give ample evidence that they were intended to be manuals for practising physicians and that they were so used. Perhaps it was because lay physicians could not be expected to be proficient in Latin that there was so much translation from Latin medical works into English. But there is equally good evidence that physicians were members of religious orders. For example, in many charm remedies the operator is told simply to sing so many psalms or litanies over the medicine and the patient, which could be done much more expertly by a cleric than by a layman. In other charms masses are to be sung

[1] *Maxims I*, 45: 'Lef man læces behoð' (*ASPR* III, 157).
[2] Such illustrations are reproduced in Grattan and Singer, *Anglo-Saxon Magic*. A physician in classical dress is shown in fig. 22 (p. 47); a physician and attendant in native dress and untonsured operating on a patient are shown in fig. 7 (p. 12), and in fig. 6 (p. 11) is shown a man in native dress, not tonsured, carrying what appear to be medicines.

over the ingredients of a medicine, which could be done only by a priest. One complicated charm text, which involves the chanting of a lorica, the writing of a cross with the oil of extreme unction and the signing of a cross on each limb of the patient is accompanied by this injunction: 'If you do not wish to do this yourself, bid the patient himself, or someone nearly related to him, and let him cross himself as well as he is able. This remedy is powerful against every temptation of the fiend.'[3] One gets the impression that the procedures may have been such as to raise doubts in the mind of a priest that it was proper for him to do them. Of course, the operator of a charm need not have been a physician, so that this caveat does not necessarily imply that an unwilling priest was also a physician. Bede also tells how Bishop John cured a young nun dying from an infected bloodletting wound in the arm, but he did this by means of prayer, not medicines.[4] Nor does Bede tell us whether the physician to whom Bishop John entrusted the treatment of a dumb lad with a scurfy head was a cleric or a layman.[5]

A few physicians are mentioned by name. There was Cynefrith, who attended St Æthelthryth of Ely in her last illness in the late seventh century, when he lanced a large tumour on her neck.[6] We do not know whether he was a member of her monastery or was called in from outside. One of the two oldest surviving Old English medical works has a colophon in Latin hexameters:

Bald owns this book, which he ordered Cild to write; earnestly here I pray all in the name of Christ that no treacherous person should take this book from me, neither by force nor by theft nor by any false speech. Why? Because no best treasure is so dear to me as the dear books which the grace of Christ attends.[7]

We do not know whether the Bald for whom this leechbook was written was a physician or not, a layman or a cleric. It is assumed that he was a physician and probably a layman who had a collection of medical works as

---

[3] *Leechdoms*, ed. Cockayne II, 350: 'Gif þe ne lyste hat hine selfne oþþe swa gesibne swa he gisibbost hæbbe 7 senige swa he selost cunne. Þes cræft mæg wiþ ælcre feondes costunge.'
[4] *HE* V.3; ed. Colgrave and Mynors, pp. 460–1.   [5] *HE* V.2; *ibid.*, pp. 458–9.
[6] *HE* IV.19; *ibid.*, p. 394.
[7] *Leechdoms*, ed. Cockayne II, 298:

> Bald habet hunc librum Cild quem conscribere iussit;
> Hic precor assidue cunctis in nomine Cristi
> Quo nullus tollat hunc librum perfidus a me
> Nec ui nec furto nec quodam famine falso.
> Cur? Quia nulla mihi tam cara est optima gaza
> Quam cari libri quos Cristi gratia comit.

the colophon attests. From the contents of his book it appears that Bald had available to him in one form or another much of the best of Byzantine and Roman medicine from the third to the ninth centuries, either in Latin or in English translation, and that he could read it well enough to order Cild to assemble it for him. It is the only Anglo-Saxon book of its kind to survive, so that we do not know whether its high standard of medical scholarship was unique or whether there were other physicians of Bald's abilities who may have commissioned similar works.

Two physicians are mentioned by name in Bald's *Leechbook*, Oxa and Dun; their names show that they were Anglo-Saxons; they must have lived no later than the ninth century. Two remedies in bk I for *þeor* are attributed to Oxa with these words: 'Oxa taught this treatment.'[8] Among the miscellaneous remedies in bk II is one beginning: 'A treatment for lung disease Dun taught.'[9] It is tempting to see in the words *lærde* and *tæhte* a reference to physicians who instructed others in their art. Is it just possible that physicians in Anglo-Saxon England trained students in medicine? A certain Baldwin was personal physician to Edward the Confessor, but his name shows that he, like so many others about Edward, was not an Englishman but was from the Continent, and so cannot count as an Anglo-Saxon physician.

Although we know so little about who the physician was or how he lived and practised his profession, we can form an estimate of his competence from his surviving writings. In Bald's *Leechbook* we find phrases which give an idea of what was expected of a practising physician. There are recipes which contain remarks such as 'as physicians know how' and 'add a sufficient amount of honey', rather than detailing the whole of the preparation of a medicine. A list of symptoms may be followed by the statement: 'Let the physician learn from this how it seems to him what should be done.' One gathers that a certain level of competence was expected of the physician. Bald's *Leechbook* also shows that at least one compiler was not a slavish copier of the masters of medicine; he often omitted parts of his sources or added to them, he re-arranged, he expressed opinions, he selected with an eye to what was important to his society, he offered substitutes for exotic drugs; in short, he behaved independently. The arrangement of his book is clear and logical, in some ways better than that of the works he drew from. We must conclude that there were

8 *Ibid.*, p. 120: 'Oxa lærde þisne læcedom.'
9 *Ibid.*, p. 292: 'Wiþ lungenadle læcedom, Dun tæhte.'

Anglo-Saxon physicians who were as able according to the conditions of their times as were any who had preceded them in the Greek and Roman world.

I have described the physician as 'he', because there is no evidence that women practised medicine. Yet it is most unlikely that Anglo-Saxon society differed in this respect from most others and that there were no women practising some form of medicine. Surely there were women midwives and village women gatherers of herbs and wise in their use and women learned in charms and amulets. But there is not a shred of evidence for their existence.

There are as few references to the physician's patients as there are to the physician himself. Three patients have already been mentioned; it is most probable that St Æthelthryth was suffering from bubonic plague when Cynefrith operated on her; if so, there was nothing he could have done except to provide relief by lancing the tumour; he could not have saved her life. Septicaemia from infected bloodletting wounds, such as the young nun suffered, must have been too common when the existence of pathogenic bacteria was unknown and infection from a dirty lancet was attributed instead to the phase of the moon or the time of day. It would be interesting to know how the physician treated the lad with the scurfy head whose speech Bishop John restored. In Bald's *Leechbook* there is a remedy for baldness:

In case one is bald Pliny the great physician gives this treatment: Take dead bees, burn to ashes and also linseed, add oil to that, cook for a very long time over coals, then strain and wring out and take willow leaves, pound, pour onto the oil, boil again for a while over coals, then strain, anoint with it after the bath. [10]

There is nothing like this in Pliny's *Historia naturalis*, but in the *Practica Alexandri* (the Latin version of the works of Alexander of Tralles) there is a similar recipe: 'That hair may not fall out but other be grown and that that which remains may be preserved: Bees are burned and mixed with oil and the hair is anointed.' [11] No such medicine is to be found in the Greek text of

---

[10] *Ibid.*, p. 154: 'Wiþ þon gif man calu sie Plinius se micla læce segþ þisne læcedom: Genim deade beon, gebærne to ahsan 7 linsæd eac, do ele to on þæt, seoþe swiþe lange ofer gledum, aseoh þonne 7 awringe 7 nime welies leaf, gecnuwige, geote on þone ele, wylle eft hwile on gledum, aseoh þonne, smire mid æfter baþe.'

[11] *Practica Alexandri*, 1v: 'Ut capilli non fluant sed alii nascantur et qui stant contineantur: Apes incendantur et misceantur cum oleo et ungantur capilli.'

Alexander, where the only ashes recommended are those of frogs.[12] Medieval cures for baldness seem to have been as strange as some recommended today, although in the case of the scurfy lad one seems to have worked better than most do today.

We have seen that Anglo-Saxon patients suffered from much the same illnesses that trouble us today, although some that our greater attention to diet and sanitation have almost banished from Western society must have been more common then. For example, because tertian malaria (*lencten adl*, 'spring fever') was endemic in the population, there are many treatments for enlargement of the spleen, and because of the presence of the parasite causing dysentery (*Entamoeba histolytica*) and of the sheep liver fluke (*Fasciola hepatica*) there are heroic treatments for abscesses of the liver. Infection of the eyes and eyelids must have been common, to judge from the numbers of remedies for them; similar evidence suggests that erysipelas and related skin infections also were common ailments as well as diseases of the throat and lungs.

For these and all the other ailments to which we are prone, the physician had little enough to offer; he could prescribe medicines, sometimes to good effect but more often giving no real medical aid. He might bleed his patients but does not seem to have employed bloodletting with the abandon indulged in later by many physicians, and his medicines seem often to have been prescribed with the knowledge that they had previously been found effective in similar circumstances. He might prescribe sensible diets, and did. Perhaps his most useful role was to offer support to his patients in the hope that recovery was possible, thus enabling them to rally their natural resources to combat their illnesses. In this he did not differ from all physicians until very recent times. Before the appearance of chemotherapeutic treatments and antibiotics (that is, before about 1930–40) there was very little in the way of medicines, apart from quinine, digitalis, morphine, aspirin and a very few others, that the physician could depend on to cure his patient; his most important role was to offer encouragement and assurance that the ailment could be overcome, and to give medicines which were often little more than placebos but which comforted the patient with the idea that something was being done for him.

[12] *Alexander von Tralles*, ed. Puschmann, p. 449: εἰσι δὲ καὶ ἀραιωτικὰ πάμπολλα, οἷον ἥ τε τῶν βατράχων τέφρα. ('There is also a large number of relaxing ones, such as the ashes of frogs').

When all else failed, the Anglo-Saxon physician could resort to charms, in themselves of no effect, but probably of great psychological benefit to the patient. All in all, if the leechbooks are a safe criterion, the Anglo-Saxon physician had access to medical works in English and to much of the post-classical Latin medical literature, which included translations and epitomes of Greek, North African and Byzantine medical authorities. He was not limited simply to a native pharmacopoeia, but could call on a wide selection of non-perishable ingredients for his medicines. His level of expertise and his attitude to medicine were impressive according to the standards of his time and his approach to medicine was predominantly rational in spite of his use of charms and magic for conditions intractable to rational treatments. Poor as Anglo-Saxon medical treatment may have been by our standards, it was probably as good as the best found elsewhere in the Western world.

4

The earliest notices of Anglo-Saxon medical practice

Apart from a few fragments, all surviving Anglo-Saxon medical texts belong to the last two centuries of the Anglo-Saxon period. Whatever we can learn about earlier medical practices, we must glean from non-medical sources. The earliest surviving writings of an Englishman are those of Aldhelm of Malmesbury, who wrote in the late seventh and early eighth centuries. In his *Enigmata* we find a few references to medicine which give a glimpse into the medical practices of his day. In *Enigma* xliii he wrote of the medicinal leech (*sanguisuga*): 'But I bite unfortunate bodies with three-furrowed wounds and so bestow a cure from my healing lips.'[1] This refers to the use of the medicinal leech to withdraw blood and perhaps to a belief that there is healing in its bite apart from its withdrawal of blood. It is interesting that nowhere in Old English medicinal texts is the bloodletting use of the leech mentioned. About the beaver Aldhelm wrote: 'Also, a healer, wounds of the entrails and limbs lurid with wasting and contagion and killing plague I disperse.'[2] *Castoreum*, which is a medically active product of the inguinal glands of the beaver, was a valued medicament in

[1] The standard edition of the *Enigmata* is in *Aldhelmi Opera*, ed. R. Ehwald, MGH, Auct. ant. 15 (Berlin, 1919), 97–149. They may also be found in *Collectiones*, ed. Glorie I, 359–540, and in translation in Lapidge and Rosier, *Aldhelm: the Poetic Works*, pp. 70–94. References to quotations from the *Enigmata* will be to the edition of Glorie. The quotation,

> Corpora uulneribus sed mordeo dira trisulcis
> Atque salutiferis sic curam praesto labellis.

from the *enigma* on the *sanguisuga* is found in *Collectiones*, ed. Glorie I, 427; trans. Lapidge and Rosier, *Aldhelm: the Poetic Works*, p. 78.

[2]
> Vulnera fibrarum necnon et lurida tabo
> Membra medens pestemque luemque resoluo necantem.

Collectiones, ed. Glorie I, 449; trans. Lapidge and Rosier, *Aldhelm: the Poetic Works*, p. 81.

ancient medicine but, so far as I know, was not prescribed for the ailments mentioned by Aldhelm, nor is it mentioned in surviving Old English remedies. On the other hand, his description of the medical uses of wallwort (*Sambucus ebulus*)[3] agrees with both Anglo-Saxon and modern herbal uses: 'From the calamities of horrible leprosy, I am able to assist them, when it vexes the viscera with corruption, that the poison may not spread, thus restoring rank entrails of men with my fruit.'[4] In the Old English medical records it was recommended for skin ailments including leprosy, and in modern herbal medicine the berries are recommended as a purgative. Aldhelm also mentions the medical uses of two other plants, but less particularly. About the greater celandine (*Chelidonium majus*) he wrote: 'If anyone should injure the eyes of my chicks, as a healer I bring a proven plaster of health, seeking a field-flower of my own name.'[5] Celandine juice was an ingredient of many collyria used for various ailments of the eyes. *Enigma* xcviii describes the physiological effects of ingestion of *elleborus*, which Aldhelm seems to have identified with what we now call woody nightshade (*Solanum dulcamara*) but which is usually thought to be one of the other drug-bearing plants of the same family, the Solanaceae.[6] It is not clear from his riddle whether the effects he describes resulted from the use of the plant as a medicine or were the poisonous effects of accidental ingestion. Although his *enigmata* were not riddles in the usual sense, his avowed aim of using them to reveal the hidden mysteries of things would have required him to choose subjects familiar to his readers and listeners, so that we may conclude that these medical references were taken from common knowledge of his day.

We have already seen that Bede's writings supply a few hints about the practice of medicine in the seventh and eighth centuries. When Cynefrith lanced the tumour on the neck of St Æthelthryth, abbess of Ely, during the

---

[3] Clapham, Tutin and Warburg, *Flora of the British Isles*. Plant names and identifications are referred to this *Flora* wherever they concern plants found in Britain.

[4] Cladibus horrendae, dum uexat uiscera tabo,
     Ne uirus serpat, possum succurrere, leprae,
     Sic olidas hominum restaurans germine fibras.

Collectiones, ed. Glorie I, 517; trans. Lapidge and Rosier, *Aldhelm: the Poetic Works*, p. 91.

[5] Si uero quisquam pullorum lumina laedat,
     Affero compertum medicans cataplasma salutis
     Quaerens campestrem proprio de nomine florem.

Collectiones, ed. Glorie I, 433; trans. Lapidge and Rosier, *Aldhelm: the Poetic Works*, p. 79.

[6] *Collectiones*, ed. Glorie I, 525; trans. Lapidge and Rosier, *Aldhelm: the Poetic Works*, p. 92.

plague of 679, the operation gave temporary relief, but the abbess died a couple of days later.[7] When Bishop John of Hexham (St John of Beverley) found that the young nun in the convent he was visiting had been bled on the fourth day of the moon he said: 'You have acted foolishly and ignorantly to bleed her on the fourth day of the moon; I remember how Archbishop Theodore of blessed memory used to say that it was very dangerous to bleed a patient when the moon is waning and the ocean tide is flowing.'[8] Theodore's warning agrees with one found in a later text: 'It is to be heeded greatly that on the fourth night of the moon or on the fifth night one should not let blood, as the books say, before the moon and sea are in agreement.'[9] But perhaps the nuns were using a bleeding chart similar to another one which survives from the late Old English period and which gives for the fourth day: 'In matutina bona est' ('It is good in the morning').[10] At any rate, we learn from this account that bleeding was practised and that bleeding charts based on phases of the moon were in use in the seventh century.

Bede's account of how Bishop John dealt with the dumb youth having a scurfy head is equally revealing; the bishop restored the lad's speech himself through prayer but also by means of a careful speech therapy which sounds remarkably modern, and turned him over to a physician for treatment of his scurfy head, so that, as Bede tells us, 'His skin was healed and he grew a beautiful head of hair. So the youth gained a clear complexion, ready speech, and beautifully curly hair.'[11] It is interesting that in this instance the bishop did not depend on prayer alone for healing, but practised a rational speech therapy and then called in a physician as well.

Bede's reference to Archbishop Theodore (above) should alert us to the possible influence of Theodore on Anglo-Saxon medicine. He was a Greek monk from Tarsus before his appointment to the see of Canterbury. Not only was he interested in medicine; he was accompanied by the African

---

[7] *HE* IV. 19; ed. Colgrave and Mynors, p. 394.   [8] *Ibid.*, pp. 460–1 (V.2).

[9] *Leechdoms*, ed. Cockayne III, 152–4: 'Is mycclum to warnienne þæt man on .iiii. nihta ealdne monan oþþe on .v. nihta menn blod ne læte swa us bec seggað ær þam þe se mona 7 seo sæ beon anræde.'

[10] This calendar of lucky and unlucky days for bloodletting is in London, BL, Arundel 60, 1r.

[11] *HE* V.2; ed. Colgrave and Mynors, p. 458–9: 'Nata est cum sanitate cutis uenusta species capillorum, factusque est iuuenis limpidus uultu et loquella promtus, capillis pulcherrime crispis.'

Abbot Hadrian, who had declined the nomination to Canterbury and had suggested Theodore instead.[12] Together these men did much to educate English students in Latin and Greek. According to Bede, some of their students (among whom were Aldhelm and Bishop John) knew Latin and Greek as well as they knew English.[13] It is possible that the later interest in Latin medicine (and Greek medicine through translation into Latin) had its inception in the stimulus given by these two men, but I can find no supporting evidence.

Bede himself in two of his works dealt directly with medical matters. A part of ch. 30 ('De aequinoctiis et solstitiis') of his *De temporum ratione*[14] is concerned with the physical and physiological fours, the relation between the four winds, four seasons and four elements of the physical world and the four ages and four humours of man. He gave as his source the *Epistula Hippocratis ad Antiochum regem*, and his text is close to those published by Helmreich and by Niedermann in their editions of Marcellus's *De medicamentis*.[15] In ch. 35 ('De quattuor temporibus, elementis, humoribus')[16] of the same work he quoted from the *Epistula Vindiciani ad Pentadium nepotem*.[17] In a more unexpected context we find a third medical reference. Some time before the completion of the *Historia ecclesiastica*, Bede revised his earlier exegetical work on the Acts of the Apostles as the *Retractatio in Actus Apostolorum*. In this revision, commenting on Acts XXVIII.8, where it is related that the father of Publius was suffering from fever and dysentery, he explained dysentery by quoting from the opening part of ch. 48 ('Ad dysenteriam') of the *De medicina* of Cassius Felix, who himself was quoting from Hippocrates.[18] It is clear from these quotations that Bede had access to one or more medical compendia. His writings make it clear that he was also familiar with the works of Pliny and Isidore of Seville, two other fertile sources of medical lore. There is no reason to suppose that other monasteries did not have access to the same or similar standard Latin works on medicine.

We know that other English monasteries also had medical texts at that

[12] *Ibid.*, pp. 328–32 (IV. 1).   [13] *Ibid.*, pp. 332–4 (IV.2).

[14] *Bedae Opera de Temporibus*, ed. Jones, pp. 235–7.

[15] Marcellus, *De medicamentis*, ed. G. Helmreich (Leipzig, 1889), pp. 5–9; also ed. Niedermann, pp. 18–35.

[16] *Bedae Opera de Temporibus*, ed. Jones, pp. 246–8.

[17] *Theodori Prisciani Euporiston*, ed. Rose.

[18] *Bedae Venerabilis Expositio Actuum Apostolorum et Retractatio*, ed. M. L. W. Laistner (Cambridge, MA, 1939), p. 145; *Cassii Felicis De Medicina*, ed. Rose, p. 122.

time. Soon after 754, Cyneheard, bishop of Winchester, wrote to Lull, bishop of Mainz, asking Lull to keep him in mind if he acquired any books on the secular sciences such as medicine, because 'we have some medical books, but the foreign ingredients we find prescribed in them are unknown to us and difficult to obtain'.[19] These medical books would have been of foreign origin; a glance at the *De medicina* of Cassius Felix, which calls for many ingredients unknown in Northern Europe, will convince one of the sort of difficulty of which Cyneheard complains. Although almost nothing of English composition has survived earlier than the reign of Alfred the Great, by that time Old English texts were being produced which prescribed not only native ingredients but others which could be obtained in England only by trade. Let us now see what some of these Anglo-Saxon medical texts were.

[19] *S. Bonifatii et Lullii Epistolae*, ed. M. Tangl, MGH, Epistolae Selectae 1 (Berlin, 1916), 247: 'Nec non et, si quos saecularis scientiae libros nobis ignotos adepturi sitis, ut sunt de medicinalibus, quorum copia est aliqua apud nos, sed tamen sigmenta ultramarina, quae in eis scripta conperimus, ignota nobis sunt et difficilia adipiscendum.' The translation is from *Bald's Leechbook*, ed. Wright, p. 30.

5

Medical texts of the Anglo-Saxons

Of the surviving medical texts demonstrably compiled by Anglo-Saxons in Old English and in Latin, the Old English ones are on the whole earlier and more voluminous than those in Latin, and for the most part are more useful for an understanding of Anglo-Saxon medical practices and beliefs. Because they are in English, we cannot suppose that they are mere 'mindless' copies of Latin sources; rather, they must have been processed through the minds of their translators and compilers, and so should give us a clearer insight into the workings of the English minds that put them together. However, Latin texts assembled by English workers are also of value for our understanding of their medicine. Almost all of those in Old English were collected by Oswald Cockayne in his *Leechdoms, Wortcunning and Starcraft of Early England*, published in three volumes in the Rolls Series between 1864 and 1866. The industry and learning of this remarkable man are truly amazing and everything done since in the field of Anglo-Saxon medicine has been done in the shadow of Cockayne's achievement.

The oldest surviving book of medicine in Old English is a beautifully made manuscript, now London, BL, Royal 12. D. xvii. It appears to have been written about 950 at Winchester and to be a copy of a lost exemplar which may have been composed about fifty years earlier in the last years of the reign of Alfred the Great.[1] It is tempting to suppose it to be a product of the literary efforts of Alfred's court, but we have not enough information to do other than guess. The manuscript is in three parts, the first two forming a single work which is usually called Bald's *Leechbook*, because of the colophon in Latin hexameters already quoted (above, p. 20) naming Bald as the owner of the book which he ordered Cild to write. We know

[1] *Bald's Leechbook*, ed. Wright and Quirk; for a discussion of the date and provenance of the manuscript, see pp. 18–23. See also *Leechdoms*, ed. Cockayne II.

nothing more of either Bald or Cild; we do not even know if Cild was the compiler of the book or simply its scribe. The third part of the manuscript, *Leechbook III*, has been overshadowed by Bald's *Leechbook*, being a much shorter and simpler compilation, but it is equally deserving of our attention, for it is the only surviving representative in Old English of the standard medical recipe book, that is, a collection of remedies with little discussion of symptoms, diagnoses or prognoses. This is a type which has survived to our own day and has a history extending back to forebears found on Sumerian clay tablets dating from the third millennium BC.

The third more or less complete collection of remedies is found in BL, Harley 585, and is known by the name *Lacnunga* ('remedies') given to it by Cockayne, its first editor.[2] It appears to be a commonplace book dating from a time somewhat later than the *Leechbooks*. Among its remedies are some of the most interesting and important of the medical charms. For the rest, *Lacnunga* shows none of the organization or medical relevance of the *Leechbooks*.

Medical recipes are also found as marginal or other additions to non-medical manuscripts. Many of them are of great interest and some are important as charms.[3] There also survives a single leaf, discovered recently, containing on one side only several remedies in Old English. This 'Omont fragment' has been dated to about 850–900 with a slight preference for a date nearer to 850 than to 900. That is, it may well be older than any other Old English medical documents, the *Leechbooks* and their exemplars.[4] It may be only a page of recipes filling part of a last leaf in a book concerned with other matters, but to me its contents suggest that it may be the last leaf of a medical compendium in which remedies were arranged in the usual head-to-foot order. This suggests in turn that there were other earlier collections similar to the surviving *Leechbooks*, of which this leaf is a lone surviving witness.

Several folios, apparently a whole quire, are missing from the Royal manuscript, so that remedies from the latter part of ch. 56 of bk II to the first part of ch. 64 of Bald's *Leechbook* are missing. This loss is particularly

---

[2] Grattan and Singer, *Anglo-Saxon Magic*; the *Lacnunga*, with translation, are on pp. 96–205.

[3] Most of these were printed by Cockayne in vols. I and III of his *Leechdoms*.

[4] B. Schaumann and A. Cameron, 'A Newly-Found Leaf', pp. 289–312; see also N. R. Ker, 'A Supplement to Catalogue of Manuscripts containing Anglo-Saxon', *ASE* 5 (1976), 121–31, at 128 (no. 417).

unfortunate, as ch. 60 (according to the table of contents) dealt with gynaecological matters, which are poorly represented elsewhere. Cockayne found on the first three folios of BL, Harley 55 medical material which corresponds in content to that given in the headnote to the missing ch. 59 of the *Leechbook*[5] and may reasonably be assumed to be a copy of it, but the rest of the missing material seems to be irretrievably lost, except for a few recipes in Nowell's transcript of the destroyed manuscript, BL, Cotton Otho B. xi.[6]

Sir Robert Cotton's library, then housed at Ashburnham House suffered severely in a fire in 1731 and Otho B. xi was almost completely destroyed. Fortunately, in 1562 Laurence Nowell had made a transcript of this manuscript and it contains a collection of medical recipes, most of which are also in Bald's *Leechbook*. Those not in the *Leechbook* as we now have it deal with ailments dealt with on its missing leaves. It is a fair assumption that they were also originally in the *Leechbook*. Because the recipes in the two collections are not quite identical, we may conclude that there were once Old English recipe books older than either.

The remaining medical documents in Old English are translations of Latin works. Of these the most important is the *Herbarium of Pseudo-Apuleius*.[7] The *Herbarium* is a complex of several works, not all dealing with plants; its origins and composition will be discussed later. This complex work was translated into English not later than the ninth or tenth century, perhaps earlier, although in its Latin form it seems to have been known in England earlier. Four manuscripts of the Old English translation survive. This relatively large number attests to the popularity of the *Herbarium* in medieval England. Because it is a translated work, its remedies cannot be considered as reflecting English practice except in so far as they can be shown to have been used by English physicians or borrowed by the compilers of other Old English works. We shall examine later the evidence for its role in Anglo-Saxon medical practice.

Of the various writings of the monk Bryhtferth of Ramsey, only a few

---

[5] *Leechdoms*, ed. Cockayne II, 280–8.

[6] London, BL, Add. 43703, 261r–264v; R. Torkar, 'Zu den ae. Medizinaltexten in Otho B. xi und Royal 12 D. xvii. Mit einer Edition der Unica (Ker, No. 180 art. 11a–d)' *Anglia* 94 (1976), 319–38.

[7] *Leechdoms*, ed. Cockayne I, 1–372. For a more recent edition (without translation) of this *Herbarium* complex together with discussion of surviving manuscripts, a copy of the Latin texts, notes and glossary, one should consult *Herbarium*, ed. de Vriend.

pages of his *Enchiridion* (written about 1011 in Old English and Latin), which contain material borrowed from Bede, and his own diagram of the relations of the microcosm (man) to the macrocosm, are of interest in the history of medicine.[8] There is also the very late *Peri Didaxeon*, found in London, BL, Harley 6258.[9] It is an incomplete translation of parts of Latin works which we will examine later. Because it appears to have been written about 1200, it is too late to be of much real value for the study of Anglo-Saxon medicine.

Works entirely in Latin are harder to assign to English origins, but at least two medical compilations in Latin are undoubtedly the work of Anglo-Saxons. They are both found in relatively late manuscripts, one in CUL, Gg. 5. 35 (the *Canterbury Classbook*), written at St Augustine's Canterbury, and entered in the manuscript about 1100,[10] and the other in Oxford, St John's College 17 (the *Ramsey Scientific Compendium*), entered at Thorney a few years later.[11] Both contain large numbers of recipes, but both also contain copies of other more general medical documents from Latin sources. From all these documents, Old English and Latin, we learn that from about 900, or earlier, to the end of the Anglo-Saxon period, the Anglo-Saxons were familiar with Latin medical texts and used them extensively.

In summary, we can say that the Anglo-Saxons had a wide acquaintance with the medical learning available in Latin; Bald and Cild and perhaps others whose works do not survive used this material together with native northern material to compile books on medicine which have the same characteristics of diagnostic and prognostic information as their Latin exemplars and which show a high level of competence in the selection and

---

[8] *Byrthferth's Manual*, ed. S. J. Crawford, EETS os 177 (London, 1929); for the diagram, see Grattan and Singer, *Anglo-Saxon Magic*, figs. 14, 15 and 16; see also below n. 10.

[9] *Leechdoms*, ed. Cockayne III, 82–144; also Löweneck, 'Peri Didaxeon', i–vii and 1–57.

[10] Only about half of the medical material in the Canterbury Classbook has been printed. The contents of the manuscript are described by A. G. Rigg and G. R. Wieland, 'A Canterbury Classbook of the Mid-Eleventh Century (the "Cambridge Songs" Manuscript)', *ASE* 4 (1975), 113–30. Two short sets of verses on medical nomenclature have been printed twice: (1) Lapidge, 'The Hermeneutic Style', pp. 67–111, at 103–5; (2) E. Jeauneau, 'Pour le dossier d'Israël Scot', *Archives d'histoire doctrinale et littéraire du moyen âge* 52 (1985), 7–71, at 20–2. About half of the remaining medical material in the manuscript has been printed as 'Das Cambridger Antidotarium' in Sigerist, *Studien und Texte*, pp. 160–7.

[11] The medical material in this manuscript is printed in Singer, 'A Review', pp. 107–60.

arrangement of their borrowed materials. The Anglo-Saxons also had a native medicine, best exemplified in *Leechbook III*, less sophisticated than that taken from Latin sources, more prone to depend on charms and other magical treatments, but nevertheless showing that this native medicine belonged to a tradition which is still transmitted in folk and herbal medicine and was competent to treat illnesses within the limitations of its period and place. The *Lacnunga* belongs to a tradition which we also have still with us: it is a compilation made by non-medical collectors, showing no evidence of arrangement or of informed choice, what we may call folk medicine at its lowest level. Consequently, in the two *Leechbook* collections, on the one hand, and in *Lacnunga*, on the other, we have examples of the two sides of the Anglo-Saxon medical world, the learned against the popular. The popularity of the *Herbarium* attests to their deep interest in medicines of plant and animal origins. And finally, compendia in Latin show that the Anglo-Saxons were familiar with most of the small treatises on diet, bloodletting, diagnosis, prognosis and so on, which formed so large a part of the common stock of Graeco-Roman post-classical medical lore.

6

Compilations in Old English

Of the three Old English medical compilations which survive in more or less complete condition, the one known as *Leechbook III* reflects most closely the medical practice of the Anglo-Saxons while they were still relatively free of Mediterranean influences. Bald's *Leechbook*, on the other hand, shows a conscious effort to transfer to Anglo-Saxon practice what one physician considered most useful in native and Mediterranean medicine. The third text, *Lacnunga*, is a sort of common place book with no other apparent aim than to record whatever items of medical interest came to the scribe's attention. In other words, of the three, *Leechbook III* can be taken to represent the oldest surviving strata of Anglo-Saxon medicine, Bald's *Leechbook* a sophisticated effort to incorporate the best of known medical practices into a physician's working manual, and *Lacnunga* a type of collection still being made by untrained and undiscriminating individuals whose chief interest to historians of medicine is that they keep alive a folk medicine which would otherwise have disappeared. We will examine them in turn, starting with *Leechbook III*.

LEECHBOOK III

If you cannot heal him with this you can never do so.[1]

Of these Old English medical texts, the oldest vernacular medical writings to survive from Western Europe, *Leechbook III* appears to be least contaminated by Mediterranean medical ideas, so that in it we come as close as we can get to ancient Northern European medicine. Consequently, it deserves

[1] *Leechdoms*, ed. Cockayne II, 328: 'Gif þu mid þys ne meaht gelacnian ne meaht þu him æfre nahte.'

close study. *Leechbook III* is almost complete; of the seventy-six chapters outlined in its table of contents, one (ch. 72: 'Wiþ attre drenc 7 smiring' ('Against poison, a potion and ointment')) does not appear in the main text; and the last two, with part of another, are lost together with the loss of a last leaf. Its arrangement follows the traditional head-to-foot order of remedies as found in almost all ancient texts: treatments for diseases and ailments of the head came first, followed by those for the eyes, the ears, the mouth, the neck and throat, the shoulders and arms, the respiratory organs, the stomach, the heart, the liver, the spleen, the abdomen, the kidneys, the urinary bladder, the lower gut, rectum and anus, the genitals, the hips, thighs, knees, shanks, ankles and feet, usually in that order. Then usually followed, in no exact order, a collection of miscellaneous remedies, which might be short but was often quite long and often contained remedies for ailments of parts of the body covered in the first part of the compilation. Up to the end of ch. 24, *Leechbook III* follows this pattern fairly closely and, for the next twenty-eight or thirty chapters, does so with many interpolations, but the last part is truly miscellaneous. That is, the book is not without order, but the order is interrupted frequently by the insertion of remedies which really belong elsewhere in the book. In this it follows the pattern of medieval books of its kind and probably reflects (to some extent) the order in which remedies were gathered for inclusion.

In it the number of remedies containing only native ingredients is high and these ingredients are usually given native English names, not Anglicized Latin ones. This implies that they are native remedies, not borrowed from Graeco-Roman cultures. The fact that the proportion of remedies which can be certainly traced to Latin texts is relatively small leads to the same conclusion. Most of those which can be traced to Latin sources or analogues are similar to ones in the *De medicamentis* of Marcellus[2] and a few others to ones in the *Herbarium*. It is important here to remember that *De medicamentis*, and to a lesser extent the *Herbarium*,[3] contain, along with much borrowed from Pliny, a great deal which is of barbarian (Gaulish) origin, so that it is possible that remedies in *Leechbook III* which seem to have come from *De medicamentis* or the *Herbarium*, may not be borrowed but are actually cognate, having come independently from a common reservoir of medicines native to Europe generally. Consequently, we may assume that *Leechbook III* gives us an insight into the barbarian past of English medicine.

[2] *Marcelli De Medicamentis*, ed. Niedermann.   [3] *Herbarium*, ed. de Vriend.

Another characteristic of the book is the relatively high proportion of magical treatments when compared with Bald's *Leechbook*. Not only are there more charms, they are usually more complex, and the number of remedies which, while not containing a charm, contain a magical component, is high. The very first remedy in the book provides an example of our conclusions so far: 'In case that one have a headache, take the lower part of crosswort [madder?], put on a red fillet, let the head be bound with it.'[4] With this compare a remedy which Marcellus gives twice: 'There is a herb or ivy which is wont to grow on any statue whatever; picked in a waning moon and bound about the head it takes away pain. If it is bound about the head or the temples tied in a red cloth with a red thread, it alleviates migraine effectively.'[5] Pliny and the *Medicina Plinii* give the same remedy.[6] That the *Leechbook* procedure is very like those recommended by Marcellus and Pliny may imply borrowing, but it may equally be the case that it comes independently from the background common to so much of medieval medicine and magic.

More indicative of common background is an amulet for the eyes: 'For swollen eyes, take a live crab, remove the eyes, and afterwards put it alive into the water, and hang the eyes around the neck of anyone who has need of them; he will soon be well.'[7] Marcellus gave the same remedy in a slightly different but also magical form: 'The eye of a crab, carefully removed and tied up in a crimson cloth and hung around the neck, is good for the early stages of bleared eyes, but only if the remedy is carried out by a

---

4 *Leechdoms*, ed. Cockayne II, 204: 'Wiþ þon þe mon on heafod ace, genim nioþowearde wrætte, do on readne wræd, binde þæt heafod mid.'

5 *Marcelli De Medicamentis*, ed. Niedermann I, 66: 'Herba uel hedera in capite statuae cuiuslibet nasci solet; ea decrescente luna sublata capitique circumligata dolorem tollit. Emigranio etiam efficaciter medetur, si in panno rufo lino rufo ligata capiti uel temporibus alligetur.'

6 *C. Plinii Secundi Naturalis Historiae Libri XXXVII*, ed. K. Mayhoff and L. Jan (Leipzig, 1875–1906), is the standard edition. The edition of bks XX–XXXII, by Jones (*Pliny, Natural History*), is more useful for the student of medical history, because of the English translation and a careful attempt to identify all plants mentioned by Pliny. The remedy is found in XXIV.170. *Plinii Secundi Iunioris qui Feruntur de Medicina Libri Tres*, ed. Önnerfors, usually quoted as *Medicina Plinii*; the remedy is on p. 8.

7 *Leechdoms*, ed. Cockayne II, 306: 'Wiþ aswollenum eagum genim cucune hrefn, ado þa eagan of 7 eft cucune gebring on wætre 7 do þa eagan þam men on sweoran þe him þearf sie; he biþ sona hal.'

chaste man.'[8] Pliny gives a similar treatment[9] and also tells of a couple of contemporary eminent Romans who sought to avoid ophthalmia by wearing around the neck an amulet consisting of a paper with Greek letters on it or a live fly tied up in a linen bag.[10] These are charms from the folk background of the people of Europe and we cannot claim that any one of them borrowed from another. We can learn something about this common folk background from a careful study of *Leechbook III*.

There are conditions which resist treatment even today. It is interesting to find that these are the ailments for which remedies most often have a magical component, as in the one for migraine given above. Warts are very intractable to treatment and one way to handle such intractable conditions was to combine the ingredients and treatments of two remedies into a single one, thereby enhancing in the patient's mind the supposed effectiveness of medicines otherwise ineffective. In Marcellus we find: 'The ashes of dog dung applied (to them) cures all kinds of warts. Also the urine of a dog with his fresh dung spread on is of very good benefit. The fresh blood of a killed mouse or the mouse itself split open and placed on heals and removes warts.'[11] The corresponding Anglo-Saxon remedy is: 'For warts take hound's urine and mouse's blood, mix together, anoint the warts with it, they will soon go away.'[12] Animal faeces were rarely prescribed in Anglo-Saxon medicine, only five times in *Leechbook III*, much less frequently than in Mediterranean medicine.

Some remedies which appear superficially to contain magic or superstitious elements will be found on closer examination to be quite rational. Before accurate time-keeping devices were available, other means for timing critical operations had to be employed. Consider this prescription:

For a carbuncle . . . make a salve: take a handful of springwort and a handful of plantain and a handful of mayweed and a handful of the lower part of dock (the kind that will swim), boil in butter, clear off the salt and the foam, add a little

---

[8] *Marcelli De Medicamentis*, ed. Niedermann I, 126: 'Cancri oculus subtiliter sublatus et in phoenicio conligatus colloque suspensus lippitudini incipienti medetur, si tamen remedium a casto homine fiat.'

[9] Pliny, *HN* XXXII.74.   [10] *Ibid.*, XXVIII.29.

[11] *Marcelli De Medicamentis*, ed. Niedermann I, 320: 'Verrucarum genera omnia fimi canini exusti cinis curat impositus. Vrina quoque canis cum suo recenti luto inlita plurimum prodest. Sanguis recens muris occisi uel ipse mus diuisus atque adpositus sanat et abolet uerrucas.'

[12] *Leechdoms*, ed. Cockayne II, 322: 'Wiþ weartum genim hundes micgean 7 muse blod, meng tosomne, smire mid þa weartan, hi gewitaþ sona aweg.'

English honey, put over the fire, boil, when it boils sing three paternosters over it, remove again, then sing the paternoster nine times over it and boil up three times and as often take it off and afterwards treat with it.[13]

The three boilings up and the three withdrawals from the fire were timed by the singing of appropriate numbers of paternosters.

It must not be thought that native Anglo-Saxon medicine was chiefly magical; most of the remedies in *Leechbook III* are rationally conceived, whether or not the treatments they recommend would be of any benefit to the patient. Many of them show good common sense, such as the advice to pregnant women to avoid salty foods, alcoholic drinks and vigorous exercise (see ch. 16). Very interesting is a treatment (incomplete) for handling a wound through which the bowels came out; the physician was to replace the bowels and then to sew up the wound with a silk suture. Silk, which would dissolve as healing took place, would not need to be removed when the wound had healed. This also shows us that silk, whether from Asia Minor or from China, was an accepted surgical necessity.

Heroic remedies were sometimes recommended: 'If a man's skull is folded up, lay the man supine, drive two stakes at the shoulders, then lay a board across his feet, then strike on it with a sledgehammer; it will come right at once.'[14] A similar treatment is found in the *Petrocellus*: 'For a folded bone in the head: lay the man out on the ground and let two men sit at the head and two at the knees and press lightly, and put a shingle at his feet and beat on that shingle with a mallet until the sick man speaks.'[15] This could well cause further damage to the brain. A group of remedies specifies salves to be applied 'in case there is a wound on top of one's head and a bone be broken and in case the shoulder stick up [i.e., be out of joint] and a good wound potion and if there be a broken bone in the head which will not

---

[13] *Ibid.*, II, 358: 'Wiþ springe . . . wyrc sealfe: nim handfulle springwyrte 7 handfulle wegbrædan 7 handfulle magþan 7 handfulle niðewearde doccan (þære þe swimman wille), [wyl] on butran, ahlyttre þæt sealt of 7 þæt fam, do hwon huniges to englisces, do ofer fyr, awyl, þonne hit wealle, sing iii pater noster ofer, do eft of, sing þonne viiii pater noster on, 7 þriwa awyl 7 swa gelome of ado 7 lacna mid siþþan.'

[14] *Ibid.*, p. 342: 'Gif men sio heafodpanne beo gehlenced alege þone man upweard, drif ii stacan æt þam eaxlum, lege þonne bred þweores ofer þa fet, sleah þonne þriwa on mid slegebytle, hio gæþ on riht sona.'

[15] London, BL, Sloane 2839, 11v–12r (*Collectio Salernitana*, ed. De Renzi IV, 195): 'Ad os plicatum in capite: Ipsum hominem ad terram extende et duo homines ad caput et duo ad genua sedeant, et premant leuiter, et ad plantas scendulam mitte et super ipsam scendulam de malliolo batis usque dum loquatur egrotus.'

come out'.[16] There are other treatments for dog and spider bites and for a thorn in the foot. These remedies all give a picture of accidents requiring medical intervention; one can envisage a fight in which a man was stabbed in the belly, a blow which broke the skull, a scrimmage in which a shoulder was wrenched out of joint and encounters with biting animals. One is saddened by the futility of the remedies. Did the man with the 'folded' skull ever recover, especially after being pounded with a sledgehammer? Of what help was a salve for a dislocated shoulder? Did the fellow with the bashed-in skull survive the removal of the pieces of bone? Was the biting dog mad? Did the spider bite or the thorn wound in the foot become septic? And what more could be done for any of these accidents? Medieval people lived in a medically dangerous and helpless world.

Not much gynaecological medicine survives; two chapters of *Leechbook III* contain most of what remains, apart from some charm material in *Lacnunga*. This material is discussed below, pp. 175–8. But one does not know into what category to place a treatment such as this one: 'Against a woman's mad behaviour: eat a radish before breakfast and that day the madness cannot bother you.'[17]

As is true for most medieval medical texts, there is very little in this *Leechbook* that can be called diagnosis or prognosis. So many remedies end with *he biþ sona hal, him bið sona sel* or words to the same effect, that one suspects them to be a sort of conventional closing rather than a firm assurance of the efficacy of the medicine. But occasionally one comes across a statement such as this following a treatment for dysentery: 'If the pottage and the drink remain inside, then you may cure the man, if they flow out, it is better for him that you do not deal with him; his fatal illness is upon him.'[18] Following the directions for making a salve for a creeping ulcer (*smeawyrm*), is the observation that: 'After they are anointed, the salve will first enlarge the wounds and eat away the dead flesh and soften the swelling and put to death the worm in it or drive it away alive and heal the

---

[16] *Leechdoms*, ed. Cockayne II, 300–2: 'wiþ þam gif man sie ufan on heafod wund 7 sie ban gebrocen 7 wiþ þam gif sio eaxl upstige 7 god dolhdrenc 7 gif gebrocen ban sie on heafde 7 of nelle'.

[17] *Ibid.*, p. 342: 'Wiþ wif gemædlan: geberge on neahtnestig rædices moran, þy dæge ne mæg þe se gemædla sceþþan.'

[18] *Ibid.*, p. 320: 'Gif se briw 7 se drenc inne gewuniað þu meaht þone man gelacnian, gif him offleogeð him bið selre þæt þu hine na ne grete; him biþ his feorhadl getenge.'

wounds.'[19] Concerning *ælfsogoþa* (an unknown ailment; Geldner suggested *elf-sucked*, that is *anaemic*[20]) this advice is given:

If one has *ælfsogoþa* his eyes are yellow where they should be red. If you wish to treat the person, consider his behaviour and observe the sex of the patient. If it is a male and he looks up when you first examine him and his face is pallid yellow, that man you might cure completely if he has not had it too long. If it is a woman and she looks down when you first examine her and her face is dusky red, you may treat her also. If it is longer by a day than twelve months and the appearance be like this, then you can improve for a while, and yet cannot cure completely.[21]

There is also a prognosis for one who is wounded: 'If a man is cut [in the flesh] and you are to treat him, see that he is facing you when you go in; then he may live. If he is turned away by no means treat him.'[22] Finally, there is a description of the appearance of one having the *wæterælfadl* ('chicken-pox', or perhaps 'measles'): 'If one has the *wæterælfadl* then his finger nails are livid and his eyes watering and he wants to look downward.'[23]

Only very rarely was there any consideration of the causes underlying the symptoms; as now with widely advertised patent medicines, treatment was for symptoms only, not for underlying causes. I find in this *Leechbook* only one example of an attempt to assign a cause to a symptom: 'For the jaundice which comes from squeezed-out bile'.[24] The recipe is also found in Marcellus, and is most likely borrowed.[25]

[19] *Ibid.*, p. 332: 'Siþþan hie gesmyred synd seo sealf wile ærest þa dolh ryman 7 þæt deade flæsc of etan 7 þone swile aþwænan 7 þone wyrm þæs on deadne gedeþ oþþe cwicne of drifð 7 þa dolh gelacnað.'

[20] Thun, 'The Malignant Elves', p. 388 (where Geldner's suggestion is noted).

[21] *Leechdoms*, ed. Cockayne II, 348: 'Gif him biþ ælfsogoþa him beoþ þa eagan geolwe þær hi reade beon sceoldon. Gif þu þone mon lacnian wille þænc his gebæra 7 wite hwilces hades hi sie. Gif hit biþ wæpned man 7 locað up þonne þu hine ærest sceawast 7 se andwlita biþ geolwe blac, þone mon þu meaht gelacnian æltæwlice gif he ne biþ þær on to lange. Gif hit biþ wif 7 locað niþer þonne þu hit ærest sceawast 7 hire andwlita biþ reade wan þæt þu miht eac gelacnian. Gif hit bið dægþerne leng on þonne xii monaþ 7 so biþ þyslicu þonne meaht þu hine gebetan to hwile 7 ne meaht hwæþere æltæwlice gelacnian.' (The manuscript has *gebetan* in the last line where Cockayne has *betan*.)

[22] *Ibid.*, p. 352: 'Gif man sie gegymed 7 þu hine gelacnian scyle, geseoh þæt he sie toweard þonne þu ingange; þonne mæg he libban. Gif he þe sie framweard ne gret þu hine ahte.'

[23] *Ibid.*, p. 350: 'Gif mon biþ on wæterælfadle þonne beoþ him þa handnæglas wonne 7 þa eagan tearige 7 wile locian niþer.'

[24] *Ibid.*, p. 314: 'Við þære geolwan adle sio cymð of seondum geallan'.

[25] *Marcelli De Medicamentis*, ed. Niedermann I, 534.

Leechbook III, then, is a relatively unsophisticated example of Anglo-Saxon medical lore in which native elements form a larger part than in either Bald's *Leechbook* or *Lacnunga* and is the closest we can get to the native medicine of the northern peoples. Its arrangement follows the pattern usual for ancient and medieval collections of remedies, but its uniqueness is that it was written in a vernacular language. Because of these characteristics, it gives us an opportunity to see European medicine at a relatively primitive level and so has a special interest for the student of the history of medicine.

BALD'S *LEECHBOOK*

Medicines for all infirmities.[26]

This treatise is an altogether different production from the one we have just considered. In the first place it is in two parts. Bk I deals with diseases whose manifestation is mostly external and arranges them more or less according to the usual head-to-foot pattern used in *Leechbook III*, but although it is in the same tradition, it is a more consciously ordered piece of work. It borrows freely from Mediterranean sources, combining them with native materials into a seamless whole. Bk II treats of internal diseases and is a thoroughly scholarly work borrowing extensively from Mediterranean sources but not subservient to them. This separation of external and internal diseases may be unique in medieval medical texts; I know of no other quite like it. The generous use of sources of Greek, Roman, North African and Byzantine origins and their blending into a harmonious whole indicate so high a level of expertise and organization that we should analyse it in some detail. As Audrey Meaney has written:

The work which resulted . . . is by far the most comprehensive and best organized of all the Old English medical compilations, and indeed . . . it must count as a very considerable achievement . . . The system used to sort and classify all this material must have been extensive and was usually also very efficient, even if some unnecessary duplications have occasionally slipped in.[27]

Joseph Payne wrote about it:

There is one book, a sort of manual for a doctor's use, of which I shall speak presently, the only surviving work of its class, which seems to imply the existence of others of the same kind. Had the single MS. which remains of this work been

[26] *Leechdoms*, ed. Cockayne II, 2: 'Læcedomas wiđ eallum untrymnessum'.
[27] Meaney, 'Variant Versions', p. 251.

destroyed, we should not know what an Anglo-Saxon professional manual was like.[28]

Because there are no surviving compilations of native medicines (except *Leechbook III*) which are older than Bald's *Leechbook*, we have very few criteria for estimating the compiler's dependence on native materials. But for remedies from Mediterranean medicine, surviving Latin compilations provide ample material for comparison. An English physician using these foreign texts was faced with the serious problem of availability of the drugs prescribed in them, which, as we have seen, prompted Cyneheard of Winchester to ask Lull to keep him in mind if he acquired any books on medicine. This problem should be kept in mind when comparing Bald's remedies with their Latin originals and when assessing which Latin texts were used as sources and which were passed over. For example, the little work of Cassius Felix from which Bede took his quotation on dysentery, in spite of its conveniently small size, had little or no influence on Old English compilations. A glance at its pharmacopoeia shows that most of its remedies, suitable for North Africa and the Mediterranean region generally, were virtually impossible to compound in Anglo-Saxon England. The same may be said for another work, the *Conpositiones* of Scribonius Largus,[29] also of slender dimensions, for which no evidence exists that it was ever used or even known in England. From works which were used the compiler made a careful selection of remedies for which ingredients were likely to be available to English practitioners.

An example of the compiler's methods can be found in a chapter from bk I; the headnote for the chapter reads:

Many and excellent medicines for a body become livid and mortified and whence the disease comes and how it should be treated if the body is so far mortified that there is no feeling in it and how the dead blood should be drawn off; and if a man's limbs should be amputated or cauterized how that should be done; pottages and potions and salves for the disease.[30]

---

[28] Payne, *English Medicine*, p. 34.

[29] *Scribonii Largi Conpositiones*, ed. G. Helmreich (Leipzig, 1887).

[30] *Leechdoms*, ed. Cockayne II, 8: 'Læcedomas micle 7 æþele be asweartedum 7 adeadedum lice 7 hwanan sio adl cume 7 hu his mon tilian scyle gif þæt lic to þon swiþe adeadige þæt þær gefelnes on ne sy 7 hu mon þæt deade blod aweg wenian scyle; 7 gif him mon lim ofceorfan scyle oððe fyr onsettan hu þæt mon don scyle; briwas 7 drenceas 7 sealfa wiþ þære adle.'

The sources may be found in *Ad glauconem Liber II*[31] and in the *Passionarius* in almost the same words. In *Passionarius* they are V.34 ('On erysipelas and its treatment'), V.35 ('On the same and its treatment')[32] and V.44 ('On gangrene').[33] The chapters on erysipelas and on gangrene are even more widely separated in *Liber II*, yet the English compiler has combined them into a single chapter. The only other place I know of where erysipelatous and erysipelas-like conditions are combined with a discussion of gangrenous conditions is in the *De medicina* of Celsus,[34] where they are also handled together. Celsus's book did not have a wide circulation; all surviving copies from the Anglo-Saxon period are continental and it is only in the arrangement of this chapter and in one or two other places in the *Leechbook* that an acquaintance with it may be hinted at. Either *De medicina* was known to the Anglo-Saxons and has left no other traces, or the compiler of the *Leechbook* recognized on his own that gangrene may be a sequela of erysipelas as well as of wounds and other injuries and combined his sources into a single account.

Material of Latin origin was used much more extensively in compiling bk II and evidences of re-arrangement and adaptation are much more obvious. For example, a long chapter on stomach ailments contains material from four chapters of its source, and the final chapter on diseases of the liver contains material from at least five different sources. Both chapters are coherent in spite of their diverse origins. In most instances where this practice of the compiler can be examined, one gets the impression that he was a practising physician who was familiar with the things he wrote about and so was drawing on personal experience when he chose treatments, and that he was careful to present them in ways designed to be most useful to other physicians. His lack of understanding is also all too evident when he discussed treatments with which he was not familiar. For example, he gave directions for the lancing of an abscess of the liver. In the account in his sources, an important part was played by a tent or wick inserted into the incision, by means of which pus and other matter could be drawn off from the abscess. This tent is not mentioned in the English translation. It is probable that the operation, which continued to be performed into the

---

[31] Cambridge, Peterhouse 251, 133r ('De cura erisipile', 'De erisipilatibus que intrinsecus fiunt'); 140v–141r ('De cancrea').

[32] *Passionarius*, 74r–v.   [33] *Ibid.*, 79r–v.

[34] *Celsus De Medicina*, ed. and trans. W. G. Spencer, 3 vols., Loeb Classical Library (Cambridge, MA, 1960–1) II, 98–106.

nineteenth century, was never done by an Anglo-Saxon physician. This might have been a good thing, as the rate of mortality was very high, probably as high as if the abscess were left alone to mature by itself.

The translation of technical medical terms from Latin into Old English must have been a major problem. Latin borrowed freely from Greek in forming its own medical vocabulary. The Anglo-Saxon writer had the choice of similarly transferring Latin and Graeco-Latin terms to English, or of finding suitable Old English equivalents. The compiler of Bald's *Leechbook* did both. His Latin was good enough that his English versions usually transmitted adequately the sense of his source; but sometimes he failed. It is easy for us, with a shelf full of reference books, to point out these errors; on the whole, given his wholly inadequate lexical aids, he did a commendable job. His success in adapting technical medical terms and in translating his sources is discussed fully below, pp. 95–9.

LACNUNGA

Here are medicines for all kinds of inflammations
and swellings and dangerous diseases.[35]

In the introduction to the edition of *Lacnunga* which he prepared with J. H. G. Grattan, Charles Singer provided a scathing assessment of Anglo-Saxon medicine: 'A.S. medicine . . . is the last stage of a process that has left no legitimate successor, a final pathological disintegration of the great system of Greek medical thought.'[36] C. H. Talbot, quoting other statements of Singer's, gave a fairer assessment of *Lacnunga*: 'The *Lacnunga* is a rambling collection of about two hundred prescriptions, remedies, and charms derived from many sources, Greek, Roman, Byzantine, Celtic and Teutonic . . . The *Lacnunga* may show "the final physiological disintegration of Greek medical thought", but it does not show that Anglo-Saxon scholars were involved in it.'[37]

Lacnunga starts out with the traditional arrangement of head-to-foot order, but before twenty remedies are entered the arrangement has been lost, the nineteenth dealing with haemorrhoids, the twentieth with the

---

[35] Grattan and Singer, *Anglo-Saxon Magic*, p. 164: 'Her syndon læcedomas wið ælces cynnes omum 7 onfeallum 7 bancoþum.'

[36] *Ibid.*, p. 94.

[37] C. H. Talbot, *Medicine in Medieval England* (London, 1967), p. 23.

preparation of oil of roses and the twenty-first with a treatment for heart attack. It looks as if the compiler may have started out with the intention of making a standard recipe book, but soon began entering things as they came to hand; no scraps of parchment for him. There is, indeed, no good reason to suppose that it ever was a planned work but that it was always a commonplace book in which things were entered higgledy-piggledy. Two scribes seem to have been involved in the making of the surviving copy;[38] the first two-thirds are in a single hand, a second hand taking over in the middle of a page. This second writer, although he entered many recipes in Old English, inserted a much larger proportion of Latin items than there are in the first part, and although the scribe (or compiler) of the first part was careless, the scribe (or compiler) of the second part was even more prone to errors.

Carelessness is a glaring characteristic of *Lacnunga*. For example, entry §94 begins: 'Here are treatments for every kind of erysipelas and inflamed sores and dangerous diseases; twenty-eight.'[39] But only thirteen are given. There were originally twenty-eight treatments for erysipelatous complaints in the group; they are all given in bk I of Bald's *Leechbook*.[40] Another entry shows mindless copying at its plainest: 'If a man's insides have a gnawing feeling: it [a plant] is called galluc dig against tearful eyes hart's horn ashes put in sweet wine the roots, pound to powder, take a good cupful, an eggshell full of wine or of good ale and honey; give to drink early in the morning.'[41] This nonsense can easily be reduced to sense. The words 'against tearful eyes hart's horn ashes put in sweet wine', are an accidental intrusion into a remedy for sore insides and for which there is an analogue in the *Herbarium* in a chapter on the uses of symphytum (i.e., galluc).[42] The recipe for tearful eyes is found in Bald's *Leechbook*, bk I.[43] Apparently in the exemplar from which the compiler (or the scribe) copied, the recipe

[38] London, BL, Harley 585, 130r–193r.

[39] Grattan and Singer, *Anglo-Saxon Magic*, p. 164: 'Her syndon læcedomas wið ælces cynnes omum 7 onfeallum [7] bancoþum eahta 7 twentige.'

[40] *Leechdoms*, ed. Cockayne II, 98–104.

[41] Grattan and Singer, *Anglo-Saxon Magic*, p. 166: 'Gif man sceorpe on þone innað galluc hatte delf wið eagena teara heortes hornes axan do on geswet win þa moran do to duste do godne cuclere fulne ægscylle fulle wines oððe godes ealað 7 hunig syle dri[n]can ær on morgen.'

[42] *Herbarium*, ed. de Vriend, p. 104; D'Aronco, 'Inglese antico *galluc*', *passim*.

[43] *Leechdoms*, ed. Cockayne II, 34: 'Gif eagan tyren, heorotes hornes ahsan do on geswet win' ('If the eyes water, put hart's horn ashes in sweetened wine').

for sore innards began at the bottom of one page and ended on the top of the next. In the bottom margin of the first page or the top margin of the second, someone wrote in the remedy for the eyes. The compiler (scribe) wrote straight through with no regard for the sense of what he was writing. But he was doing no worse than his modern editors; Cockayne, Leonhardi, and Grattan and Singer supposed the confusion to have arisen from an omission rather than an addition although the means for correction were available to them. These two examples illustrate the lack of understanding of his material which characterizes the compiler of *Lacnunga*.

But we must not be too hard on him. Precisely because he was inattentive and ignorant, a great deal of interesting material got past him and was recorded in his commonplace book. Consequently, we find in it two outstanding pagan charms, one for sudden stitch caused by the assaults of witches, elves and Æsir,[44] the other for *dweorh*,[45] a fever with delirium. There are also other charms of Teutonic origin, ones from Ireland and ones which are purely Christian. It is invaluable as a source of superstitious medicine, and although it nowhere reflects the best in Anglo-Saxon medical practice, it gives a fascinating insight into its less rational aspects.

[44] Grattan and Singer, *Anglo-Saxon Magic*, pp. 172–6.   [45] *Ibid.*, pp. 160–2.

7

Compilations in Latin

If you wish to be an accomplished physician,
always be cautious and you will not be at fault.[1]

Some medical ideas and theories common to the Mediterranean world, such
as that of the four humours and the practice of bloodletting to keep them in
balance, or the role of dieting in preserving and restoring health, although
practised assiduously by the Greeks and Romans and their followers, do
not seem to have received as much attention from the Anglo-Saxons. But
that they were acquainted with these theories and practices is clear from
medical collections in Latin made by the Anglo-Saxons. We will find it
useful to examine these to find out what an Anglo-Saxon physician might
be expected to know about the best-established theories of disease and
treatment in medieval Europe.

Medical collections in Latin of undoubted Anglo-Saxon compilation are
obviously not as easy to identify as Old English ones, but at least two such
survive in fairly late manuscripts, one in the *Canterbury Classbook* (CUL,
Gg. 5. 35)[2] and the other in the *Ramsey Scientific Compendium* (Oxford, St
John's College 17),[3] both of about 1100. There are other smaller texts,
mostly of the kind Cockayne called 'flyleaf leechdoms'. All these give a
picture of medical lore of Mediterranean origin available to the Anglo-
Saxons independently of the *Leechbooks* and *Lacnunga*. They show that

---

[1] CUL, Gg. 5. 35, 427r: 'Si vis perfectus esse medicus semper time et non culpaberis.'

[2] *Ibid.*; the two sets of verses in hexameters on medical terminology are on 422v–423r, the
remaining material on 425–430r and 445v–446v (copied by a different and later scribe).

[3] Oxford, St John's College 17, 1v–2v and 175r–177v. See Singer, 'A Review',
pp. 107–60.

Englishmen were acquainted with most of the minor works which circulated freely, usually pseudonymously or anonymously, through the whole of the Middle Ages. A summary of their contents shows that they were often of dubious medical value.

THE *CANTERBURY CLASSBOOK*

The *Canterbury Classbook* contains, in fact, two separate texts. One consists of two short sets of hexameter verses on medical terminology (423r–v), and the other is a long incomplete collection of the minor works just mentioned together with more than 200 recipes (425r–430r and 444v–446v). The two sets of hexameter verses are interesting because they show that Anglo-Saxons were anxious to retain and understand medical terms of Greek origin, just as today most medical terms are derived from Greek. The first little poem is in the form of a challenge to the auditor (reader) to identify twenty-seven medical terms. The opening in two lines borrowed from Alcuin encourage him to identify them. 'Tell me two nouns which provide synonyms for all (the following terms); tell all things about each word, what every syllable signifies.'[4] The last line reads: 'If you do not explain them, you will go away unrewarded.'[5] This sounds like an examination set for students; it is accompanied by a set of glosses for each word in what would appear to be a master's crib.

The glosses, and the words to be identified, are taken from the *Quaestiones medicinales*, whose source is a Greek work, the Ὅροι ἰατρικοὶ, wrongly attributed to Galen. Only two incomplete copies of the *QM* survived to our time, one in the British Library, and the other in the Bibliothèque Municipale at Chartres, where it was destroyed during the Second World War.[6] The date of the poem is uncertain; it survives in three manuscripts, the oldest being of the eighth or ninth century. It may well date from the Canterbury school of Theodore and Hadrian in the late seventh century.

The second poem is in some ways more of a challenge to modern students

---

[4] Lapidge, 'The Hermeneutic Style', p. 103: 'Dic duo que faciunt pronomina nomina cunctis,/ Omnia dic que sunt uerba que silliba signet.'

[5] 'Si non exposueris indonatus abibis.'

[6] M. L. Cameron, 'Some Greek Medical Terms known to the Anglo-Saxons', *ASE* (forthcoming). The *Quaestiones medicinales* were edited from London, BL, Cotton Galba E. iv (s. xiii) by Rose, *Anecdota Graeca* II, 243–74, and (in part only) from Chartres, Bibliothèque Municipale, 62 (s. x^{ex}) by Stadler, 'Neue Bruchstücke', pp. 361–8.

because it is not glossed, a challenge at least equal to that given to medieval ones. It consists of forty-seven medical terms arranged in ten hexameter verses; the last word is 'tricocinare' ('sift it out (for yourself)'). Lapidge recognized a medical glossary published by Goetz from two manuscripts (one tenth century, the other from the early eleventh) as a source of most of its words.[7] The remainder can be found in Isidore's *Etymologiae* and in *Petrocellus* (or its sources). The 'poet' was obviously trying to set out forty-six Greek medical terms in Latin script; he included a couple of Latin ones; his spelling and that of his sources show that their grasp of Greek was minimal or non-existent. The most that can be said for these two sets of verses is that they show a continuing interest on the part of Anglo-Saxons in classical medical terminology, an interest which must have been most useful, as the Latin texts with which they were familiar continued to use Greek medical terms as frequently as Latin ones.

The remaining medical material in the *Canterbury Classbook* was entered later than the main text, on leaves at the ends of two sections, but apparently forms a single compilation which is incomplete owing to the loss of the last quire(s) of the manuscript. Sigerist printed the first part as the *Cambridger Antidotarium*, a misleading title, as most of the material is not an antidotary proper.[8] It is worthwhile enumerating its various parts as they show the sort of thing which circulated all over Europe wherever medical collections were made. The first item (425r) deals with the procedure to be followed during a regimen of purging the bowels; it is taken from a collection known as the *Sorani Ephesii uetustissimi archiatri et peripatetici, in artis medendi isagogen*, of which no manuscripts survive, it being known only from a printed version made at Basel in 1528.[9] This collection is a pseudonymous work, having no known connection with the true works of Soranus, but the material of its twenty-three chapters had a wide circulation in the Middle Ages.

The second item (425v–426r) is a small tractate on bloodletting, purging and dietary regimen which quite early was attributed to Bede, but is now included among his pseudonymous works.[10] Although it has no

---

[7] See Lapidge, 'The Hermeneutic Style', pp. 84–5 and 104–5.

[8] *Studien und Texte*, pp. 160–7.

[9] *Sorani Ephesii Vetustissimi Archiatri et Peripatetici, in Artis Medendi Isagogen*, ed. A. Thorin (Basel, 1528).

[10] *Bedae Pseudepigrapha, Scientific Writings Falsely Attributed to Bede*, ed. C. W. Jones (Ithaca, NY, 1939); PL 90, 959–62.

known direct source, the advice it gives is similar to that in other medieval tractates on the same subjects. It is followed by a small item (426r) on the signs of death, wrongly attributed to Galen. With it is a tiny article on urinoscopy as a prognosis of death or disease by examination of the patient's urine. The whole passage is worth quoting:

Galen says: What signs of death appear in the human body? The brow becomes red, the brows slacken, the left eye becomes smaller, the tip of the nose becomes white, the chin falls, the pulse runs ahead, the feet are cold, the belly shrinks, a young person is sleepless, an old one sleeping. Urine dark in the morning is very bad. Urine pure and cloudy signifies approaching death. Red urine if it has sediment is not dangerous. Urine white in the morning, clear again after breakfast is best.[11]

I know of no direct sources for the prognostics in this little tract, but the first part resembles to some extent material in Hippocrates's treatise Προγνωστικόν[12] and most of the information on prognosis from urines can also be found in the same treatise.

The next item (426r–v) is another well-known one dealing with bloodletting and diet for each month of the year. It also is found in the pseudo-Soranus and in *Petrocellus*; its form here is so like that of the *Petrocellus* entry that it may well have been copied from it. A fragment of a treatise follows (426v–427r), on the four humours and their relations to the parts of the body and the seasons of the year; it is known as the *Dialogus Platonis et Aristotilis* and was widespread in medical literature. Next, from the *Isagoge* and *Petrocellus* is an entry (427r) describing the various veins used in bloodletting, their locations and the ailments for which blood is let from them, each vein being responsible for a certain part of the body and its ailments. The next item (427r–v) continues the subject of bloodletting by outlining the advantages which it confers on the body and goes on to outline the treatments to be applied when infection or other harm follows bloodletting. There are directions concerning the amount of blood to

[11] 'Dicit Galienus: In humano corpore que signa mortifera apparent? Frons rubet, supercilia declinantur, oculus sinister minuitur, nasi summitas albicat, mentum cadit, pulsus ante currit, pedes frigescunt, uenter defluit, iuuenis uigilans, senex dormiens. Urina nigra mane pessima est. Urina pura et nebulosa proximam mortem significat. Urina rubra si habuerit fecem non periclitabitur. Urina mane alba, post prandium rursus candida optima est.' See also V. Nutton, 'Prognostica Galieni', *Medical History* 14 (1970), 96–100.

[12] E. Littré, *Œuvres complètes d'Hippocrate* II, 110–91.

remove depending on its appearance when it first flows. One realizes the dangers of this kind of therapy when one reads:

Do not let blood run so long that lipostomia occurs, that is, weakness and infirmity of the stomach. Because if the body is chilled by emission of blood, on that account bile ascends in the brain, or phlegm is locked up in the stomach, having no exit. Because if proper blood is drawn that is harmful; if deleterious is drawn, that helps. And if lipostomia occurs do this diligently: In winter foment the feet and face with hot water, in summer with cold.[13]

The weak grasp of Greek terminology is evident in the word 'lipostomia', which stands for λιποθυμία ('swooning', 'fainting') and which Cassius Felix transliterated as 'lipotomia'. If we add to the dangers of swooning from loss of blood those of difficulty in stopping haemorrhage from an incised blood vessel and of infection of the wound, bloodletting must have been a therapy of most doubtful utility. It is incredible that it continued to be used in medicine into the late nineteenth century.

The last item on bloodletting (427v) discusses treatments to be carried out in various months by letting blood for various ailments. It is worth quoting, because it shows how gratuitously bloodletting was carried out as a sort of prophylaxis:

It is good to take precautions in certain months, as many authors have written. In April lance the median vein of the arm for trouble with the chest and liver, in September the lateral vein for pleurisy and liver ailments. In November it is good to apply cupping glasses with scarifications, because at that time all the humours are ready. In December lance the cephalic vein for ailments of the head and for watering of the eyes. In February lance the vein in the thumb because then the earth is sick with fever, and everything that is in it.[14]

[13] CUL, Gg. 5. 35, 427v: 'Non tamdiu currat sanguis ut lipostomia fiat, id est, lassitudo uel debilitatio stomachi. Quia si emissione sanguinis infrigidat corpus, pro hoc colera ascendit in cerebro, aut flegma nimia conclusa est in stomacho, non habens exitum. Quia si sanguis proprius tollatur, nocuum est; alienum si tollatur, adiuuat. Et si lipostomia contingit, talem facies diligentiam: Hiemis tempore, plantam pedis et faciem ex calida aqua fouebis, ⟨aestate ex frigida⟩.' (The last three words are missing from the manuscript.)

[14] *Ibid.*, 427v: 'Bonum est per singulos mensis dies habere studium, sicut multi autorum scripserunt. Aprili mense, uenam medianam de brachio incide, pro torace et pulmonis causa; mense Septembri uenam lateranam propter pleuresin et epaticis. Mense Nouembri bonum est garsis uentosas inponere, quia in ipso tempore sunt omnes humores parate. Mense Decembri uenam cefalicam incide propter capitis uitia et oculorum infusionem. Mense Februario uenam de pollice incide quia tunc febricitat terra et omnia que in ea sunt.'

The remainder of these materials (427v–431v and 444v–446v) consists of some 246 entries, of which two are taken from the pseudo-Soranus, chs. 20 and 11, respectively. One of these (429v) is a medicine to be taken throughout the year; beginning in March one is to drink a potion containing pepper, cloves, pelletory of Spain, honey and strong wine, to be taken fasting or after eating throughout the whole of the month. In each following month one or more extra herbs is to be added to the potion. If carefully followed this regimen was supposed to keep the head and breast and all the internal organs from harm, prevent superfluities and dry up humours. The other (430v) is a short disquisition on the advantages of frequent vomiting; one who vomits frequently should always be healthy, because vomiting removes bile and phlegm which harm the head and it also prevents the illnesses which come from overeating and poor digestion. The remainder of the group are short recipes in no obvious order giving medicines for all sorts of ailments.

Of the 246 entries the last seven are not simple recipes. The first of these is a virtually complete copy (446r) of the *Epistula Vindiciani ad Pentadium nepotem*, which we found Bede quoting from. In this much-quoted letter, Vindicianus gave his nephew a short lesson on the humours and their roles in human health and disease during the four seasons of the year, their influence on the characters of men, and the need for physicians to be cautious in their use of bloodletting and how humours may be controlled and an ailing person restored to health by careful attention to diet. The remaining six entries (446v) are taken from *Petrocellus*, and deal with paralysis, frenzy, stroke, epilepsy, fevers, etc. The last of them is a mere fragment, the remainder lost with the rest of the manuscript.

I have not made a detailed study of source/analogues of the recipes in the collection, chiefly because most medical Latin recipe collections are unpublished and available for study only with difficulty. A few of its recipes are analogous to ones in Marcellus, and many of them are similar to ones which turn up in late medieval English collections such as that in the Thornton manuscript edited by M. Ogden.[15] Their ingredients show that most of them belong to a Mediterranean background.

[15] *Liber de Diversis Medicinis*, ed. M. Ogden, EETS os 207 (London, 1938).

The second large collection, on the first two and last three folios of the *Ramsey Scientific Compendium* (1v–2v and 175r–177v), by their position in the manuscript cannot be part of the original compilation which may be dated to 1110–1111.[16] The first item (1v) is an extract from the *Epistula Vindiciani ad Pentadium nepotem*, already described. It deals with the qualities of the four humours and their sites in the body. It is followed by another longer one (1v) also on humours, source unknown, and also found in the *Canterbury Classbook*. Then a short paragraph, source unknown (1v), on the necessity to purge at certain times of the year to maintain humoral balance. Two long sections on bloodletting, found also in *Petrocellus* and containing material similar to that in the *Canterbury Classbook*, complete a quite long discussion on humours (1v–2v), their role in health and disease and the function of bloodletting and diet in keeping them in balance.

These are followed by the same prognostics of death (2v) as discussed above (p. 51), a long list of plant names with glosses and one dealing with weights and measures. An unusual extra prognostic is given: 'That you may learn if a sick person will live: smear his hand with leaven, then give it to a dog to eat; if he eats it, he will live, if not, he will die.'[17] A number of electuaries (sweetened medicines to be licked from a spoon), a paragraph on dangerous days and a number of remedies, all from unidentified sources, for various ailments, complete the medical material on the first two folios of the manuscript.

The material on the last folios (175r–177v) begins with a number of recipes, mostly unidentified, and, in the margin of 175r, a charm for nosebleed and a short article on the various kinds of fevers and their causes. As this latter contains most of the ideas about fevers current in the Middle Ages, it bears quoting:

Quotidian fever comes from phlegm, tertian from red bile, quartan from melancholic, that is, black bile. Simonacus [this may be a mistake for 'simplex', simple] is ephemeral, arising daily from blood [the text here is corrupt]. Synochal is continually in fever. Quotidian comes from cold humour, because phlegm is cold and moist. Tertian from hot, because red bile is hot and dry. Quartan from

---

[16] M. Lapidge, 'A Tenth-century Metrical Calendar from Ramsey', *Revue Bénédictine* 94 (1984), 326–69, at 348–50.

[17] Singer, 'A Review', p. 133: 'Ut scias si possit uiuere infirmus: Fermento manus eius illinias, postea da cani manducare; si manducauerit, uiuet, si non, morietur.'

melancholy, because it is dry and cold. Simonacus from blood because it is hot and moist. So when there is a quotidian fever, give cold food before the paroxysm. But during the paroxysm give him nothing, but before the paroxysm give him pottage having pepper and cumin and feet of suckling veal well cooked and well seasoned with vinegar and honey and pennyroyal and buns of fine wheaten flour having a bit of oil, and if he is filled, make for him water and with it root of celery, fennel and parsley and give it to him to drink.[18]

Here we find in this single article the theory that disease (here various forms of malaria) is caused by imbalance of one of the four humours with the idea that each humour has two of the four qualities of heat, moisture, dryness and cold. There is the usual attention to a diet designed to counteract the qualities of the humour responsible for the fever, and the starving of the fevered patient, a treatment that still survives in the injunction to 'feed a cold and starve a fever'. Moreover, because a quotidian fever is due to phlegm, which is cold and moist, the foods recommended to be taken before onset of the attack are neutral (the pottage and veal feet), but seasoned with other ingredients all of which are hot and dry, the idea being that the effects of the phlegm may be counteracted by the contrary properties of the seasonings. This theory of the temperament of foods controlling the temperament of the eater had wide acceptance in medieval times. For instance, Charlemagne in his last years complained that his doctors insisted on his eating boiled meats rather than the roasted ones he preferred.[19] Anglo-Saxon physicians do not seem ever to have embraced fully this concept of adjusting diet by means of seasonings and manner of cooking in order to control the humoral balance of the body; at least, it

---

[18] *Ibid.*, p. 138: 'Cotidiana febris sit ex fleumate, tertiana ex colera rubea, quarta ex melancolico id est nigro colere. Simonacus est effemerus, ex sanguine cotidana omnibus sit res(?) accensa. Sinocus semper febrens est. Cotidiana sit ex frigido humore, quia fleuma frigus et humida est. Terciana ex calido, quia colera rubea calida et sicca est. Quartana ex melancolico, quia siccus et frigidus est. Simonacus ex sanguine quia calidus et humidus est. Cum igitur febris cotidiana fuerit, cibum dabis calidum ante accessionem. In accessione autem nichil dabis ei, sed ante accessionem dabis ei pulcinum manducare habentem piper et cuminum et pedes lactantis pecudis bene coctos et bene conditos de aceto et melle et pulegio, et bucellas de silicino habentes modicum oleum, et si satierit fac ei aquam eoquam radice apii, feniculi ac petrofolii et da ei bibere.'

[19] *Einhard's Life of Charlemagne*, ed. H. W. Garrod (Oxford, 1925), p. 25: 'Et tunc quidem plura suo arbitratu quam medicorum consilio faciebat, quos paene exosos habebat, quod ei in cibis assa, quibus assuetus erat, dimittere et elixis adsuescere suadebant.'

does not appear in Old English documents and the reasoning behind the directions may not have been appreciated when encountered in texts such as this one.

The next item (175v–176r) is a version of the *Epistula Hippocratis ad Maecenatum*, another pseudonymous work of wide circulation in the Middle Ages. It also deals with the association of four parts of the human body (head, breast, belly, bladder) with the four seasons, the four properties of matter and the four humours. Singer, not recognizing its origin, entitled it 'On the principles of pathology' and added:

The passage . . . is of interest as the only known Western attempt of that period to explain in detail the origin and cause of disease. A century or so later such attempts are not uncommon, but in Western Europe, in the first few years of the twelfth century, this passage stands alone. It is probably taken either from a Salernitan writer or else from Constantine.[20]

I do not know how old it is, but it is found in ninth-century manuscripts and so is centuries older than either Constantinus Africanus (*c.* 1020–87) or the Salernitan School. Singer was convinced that no rational thought appeared in medieval medicine before the influence of the Arabs was propagated by Constantinus and his successors. The text itself is too long to be quoted entire but a single short extract will show its origins: 'When blood is abundant it brings about illness and from it arises sanies [corrupted blood and humours], which is seen in cut wounds.'[21] The theory that blood, having left the blood vessels, became corrupt and formed pus was a cornerstone of Hippocratic medicine, and there was an elaborate theory of how it could leave the vessels under the influence of various things causing 'spasms' and so lead to suppurating wounds. Other ideas in the *Epistula* can also be traced back to the teachings of the Hippocratic school and to Galen, although as a whole it is an independent composition.

The remainder of the medical entries are recipes (176r–177v). Of these recipes, the first group is arranged as a sort of short herbal, with plant names given in alphabetical order followed by brief statements of their medical uses; for example 'Heliotrope, that is, solsequia: the juice gets rid of poison, its leaves pounded cure dislocations, taken in food it is good for

[20] Singer, 'A Review', pp. 156–7.

[21] *Ibid.*, p. 140: 'Sanguis cum habundat ualitudinem infert et ex ea nascitur sanies, quam in uulneribus sectis uidetur.'

the stomach.'[22] Apart from a few found also in Marcellus and Pliny, these recipes have not been traced to source/analogues. Two of them, however, deserve mention: 'Enema sciaticis . . . addens furfuras triticeas galoxinas .ii. . . . tepidum inicias' and 'Enema ad eos . . . furfuribus triticeis galoxinas .ii. . . . tepidum inicias.'[23] These are variants of a remedy found elsewhere in the period we are dealing with in the *Liber Teropetici* (*Teraupetica*) of Northern Italian provenance. The word 'galoxina', meaning 'double handful' is very rare in the medical literature and its use here leads to unresolved speculations about the source of recipes in the collection in the *Ramsey Compendium*.

Because Singer's is still the only printed version of this important collection, and because he has expressed ideas concerning it which are not now considered valid, I should like to draw attention to the more erroneous of these ideas. In the *Epistula Hippocratis* quoted in the collection, potions are recommended against all onsets of diseases. Singer calls these potions a panacea and claims that they are due to Arab influence, because (he said) it is well known that panaceas first appeared in Europe in the eleventh century. But the *Epistula* was current in the ninth. Again, one of the 'recipes' of the collection gives directions for catching birds: 'That you may take birds by hand. Macerate grain in lees of wine, mix the lees with hemlock juice and scatter for the birds. If any of them tastes it, it will not fly.'[24] Singer wrote:

We will terminate our list of recipes with our author's version of that method of catching birds which so puzzled our childhood. It serves at least to illustrate how low the intellect had fallen in that age. 'To capture birds in the hand. Macerate cheese in the lees of wine, mix the lees with the juice of hemlock and sprinkle on the birds. If one of them tastes it, he will be unable to fly.'[25]

It was Singer who salted the birds' tails, not the recipe-maker with the 'low intellect' who apparently knew the toxic effects of hemlock (*Conium maculatum*) well enough to use it to stun birds. It is dangerous to impute low intellect to a society which could produce an Aldhelm, a Bede, an Alfred, a Dunstan, an Ælfric or a Bald; within the limitations of their

---

[22] *Ibid.*, p. 143: 'Eliotropia, id est solsequia, sucus uenenum extergit, folia eius tunsa luxum sanant, in cibo sumpta stomacho prodest.'

[23] *Ibid.*, p. 146: see also *Liber teropetici*, in London, BL, Arundel 166, fol. 32r.

[24] *Ibid.*, p. 148: 'Vt aues manu capias. Frumentum in fece uini macerabis; feces dico mixtas cum suco cicute et auibus sparge. Si quis inde aliquid gustauerit, non uolabit.'

[25] *Ibid.*, p. 159.

training they show intellect of as high an order as any other society has produced.

It is impossible to say what part, if any, Anglo-Saxons played in the compilation of other medieval Latin medical works, such as the *Petrocellus*, which bears a striking resemblance in its composition to Bald's *Leechbook*, and may very well be a product of an Anglo-Saxon physician. There is ample proof from surviving Latin and Old English medical texts that Latin medical literature was as well known in England as elsewhere in Europe and that it was intelligently studied and used. But the most that can be said at this time is that, while Bald's accomplishment is unique among vernacular medical texts, there was at least one Latin compilation assembled according to the same plan.

8

Latin works translated into Old English: *Herbarium* and *Peri Didaxeon*

Therefore it seems better to me – if it seems so to you – that we too should turn into the language that we can all understand certain books which are most necessary for all men to know.[1]

Two Latin works of considerable length which were known to the Anglo-Saxons from fairly early times – the *Herbarium of Pseudo-Apuleius* and its associated works (the *Herbarium* complex or *Herbarium*, for short) and the *Petrocellus* – were eventually translated into Old English, the latter only in part and at a very late date.

HERBARIUM COMPLEX

The *Herbarium* complex contains several works: a group of works giving medicines derived from plants, followed by other, shorter, ones giving medicines derived from animals. The Old English translation of this complex must have met a real need; four copies survive, one of them (London, BL, Harley 6258B, of about 1200) having the herbs arranged in alphabetical order according to their Latin names. There is also evidence that the Latin version was known in England from the eighth century and probably earlier. The oldest surviving manuscript (BL, Harley 585, which also contains *Lacnunga*) was written about 1000, so that the text may be as

---

[1] King Alfred's preface to his translation of Pope Gregory's *Regula pastoralis*, trans. S. Keynes and M. Lapidge, *Alfred the Great. Asser's Life of King Alfred and other Contemporary Sources* (Harmondsworth, 1983), p. 126. Although Alfred did not have medicine in mind when he made his translations, his reasons apply equally well to the translations of medical works into Old English.

much as a century later than Bald's *Leechbook*, but, as the language shows the characteristics of West Saxon, the translation may belong to the same school which produced the *Leechbook*.[2]

Like its Latin exemplars, the Old English version contains several works: (1) a short treatise on the medical uses of betony, ascribed in the Latin versions to Antonius Musa and separate from the *Herbarium* proper, but anonymous in the English one and numbered continuously with it; (2) the *Herbarium* proper, ascribed to an otherwise unknown Apuleius Platonicus, but not separately identified in the English version; (3) a supplementary herbal usually ascribed to Dioscorides in the Latin versions but written continuously with the first in the English one. In the Old English version these three treatises are written throughout as a single work with continuous chapter numbering and a single table of contents, whereas in the Latin manuscripts the supplementary herbal usually ascribed to Dioscorides is a separate work, in some manuscripts immediately following the main herbal, in some following the *Medicina de quadrupedibus*. It is supposed that the Old English translation followed a version in which the three herbal treatises were together. The *Medicina de quadrupedibus* in the English version (the name was given to it by Cockayne in his edition but is not found in any extant manuscripts), is also a composite collection consisting of (1) a short treatise on the medical uses of a badger, in the form of a letter sent by the otherwise unknown Egyptian king Idpartus to the Emperor Octavian; (2) an anonymous treatise on the healing properties of the mulberry, which, although it mentions no animal, is included in the *MDQ*; (3) a version of the *Liber medicinae ex animalibus* (ascribed in the Latin versions to a certain Sextus Placitus) giving medicines using products derived from twelve wild and domestic animals. In the Old English translation these three treatises are numbered as a single work.

There are two extant versions of the Latin *Herbarium* complex. They differ particularly in that one contains what de Vriend calls the A-version of the *MDQ* and the other the B-version; also the supplementary herbal in one is the *Liber medicinae ex herbis femininis* (EHF), and in the other it is the *Curae herbarum* (CH).[3] Not all versions contain the treatise on the mulberry, but it is usually found in those versions which also contain the

---

[2] *Herbarium*, ed. de Vriend. See the Introduction, pp. xi–lxviii, for references to the contents of this and the next paragraphs.

[3] W. Hofstetter, 'Zur lateinischen Quelle des altenglischen Pseudo-Dioscurides', *Anglia* 101 (1983), 315–60.

A-version of the *MDQ* and the *CH* version of the supplementary herbal. The Old English translation follows the A-version of the *MDQ*, has the treatise on the mulberry and in its supplementary herbal material has nine chapters found in *CH* only (not in *EHF*); the remainder are found in both *CH* and *EHF* or in *EHF* only. Either the Old English supplementary chapters are a selection from both herbals or the translation was made from a Latin manuscript which has not survived in which the selection had already been made. Although both *EHF* and *CH* show strong similarities to Dioscorides, neither is taken directly from his works and both contain chapters on herbs not dealt with by him, so that it is not correct to claim, as Cockayne did, that the Old English herbal supplement is taken from Dioscorides.

Of the four surviving Old English manuscripts, only one (BL, Cotton Vitellius C. iii) is illustrated; its illustrations are very similar to those of a ninth- or tenth-century manuscript from Montecassino (Montecassino, Archivio della Badia, v. 97), and are of plant species found around the Mediterranean, although the majority of them were also to be found in England. The English rubricator apparently followed his exemplar closely. He used a green pigment which has had disastrous results for the manuscript; wherever it was applied, it has eaten away most of the vellum leaving holes, so that what was once an elegant manuscript has now a rather moth-eaten appearance. In the Ashburnham House fire in 1731, the top edges of the leaves were scorched and have shrunk and cracked, distorting the writing on the upper two or three lines. In spite of these accidents, the book still shows the care with which it was made. It must have been considered a work of much importance to warrant such attention to its production. The text of Hatton 76 in the Bodleian Library is produced in exactly the same two-column format as the Cotton manuscript but the spaces left for illustrations have not been filled in. In Harley 585 no provision was made for illustrations. The remaining manuscript, Harley 6258B, is best described in Cockayne's words: 'MS O is a mean manuscript.'[4] At one time it also suffered damage, probably from fire; its date after the Norman Conquest makes it too late for serious consideration within the context of the present discussion.

The texts of all four manuscripts derive from a single translation and may be considered as a unit for our purposes. As the Cotton manuscript is

---

[4] *Leechdoms*, ed. Cockayne I, lxxxiv.

the only one illustrated, we will take it, as did Cockayne and de Vriend, as the primary one for study. Because it is a translation and not an original compilation, we cannot analyse it in the same way as we will the *Leechbooks* and *Lacnunga*; rather, we will concentrate on the competence of the translator to handle his Latin text and to identify its plants and animals. We can also look at some of the alterations he made in the arrangement of his text and at some of his omissions from it. We can also examine the illustrator's ability to identify his plants.

On the whole, the translation is correct. There are occasional mistakes which completely change the intent of a recipe such as in ch. 18, where the translator rendered *ad caput deplendum* ('for purging the head') by *wið þæt mannes fex fealle* ('in case one's hair is falling out'), thus changing a remedy for clearing the head into one to prevent falling hair by reading *deplendum* ('emptying') as if it were *depilendum* ('removing the hair'). He repeated the mistake in ch. 21, so that we probably should not attribute it to an error in his exemplar.[5] Evidently he did not know the meaning of the word *chironius* ('chronic', of long standing and difficult to heal) because in ch. 9 he did not translate it, and in ch. 23 did translate *ad vulnera cyronia* ('for chronic ulcers') by *wið handa sare* ('for sore hands');[6] Cockayne probably guessed correctly when he assumed that the translator associated *cyronia* with χείρ ('hand') rather than with the centaur Chiron.[7] Ch. 89 of the Latin version gives as the ingredient of a recipe *herbae rubi aut flos aut mora* ('bramble flower or berries'); the translator took *mora* to mean *delay* rather than *berries* and wrote *genim þysse sylfan wyrte blostman . . . butan æclre ydincge* ('take blossoms of this same herb . . . without any delay').[8] He sometimes had trouble with technical terms, as in ch. 4 of *MDQ*, where he translated *alopitias* ('fox-mange', in which hair falls out) by *heafodsare* ('pain in the head').[9] In ch. 2.15 of the *Herbarium*, he had trouble with *secundarum* ('of the afterbirth'); this remedy follows closely a couple for fevers (no. 12 for quartan and no. 14 for tertian) and he assumed that *secundarum* also referred to a fever, *þe ðy æftran dæge to cymeð* ('that comes on the second day'), i.e., a quotidian.[10] In chs. 3 and 12 of *MDQ* he misunderstood the word *moium, mugium* ('penis') and translated it by *scytel* ('excrement', 'dung'); in fact, he did so poor a job of 3.14 that the scribe of

[5] *Herbarium*, ed. de Vriend, pp. 62–3 and 68–9. [6] *Ibid.*, pp. 52–3 and 70–1.
[7] *Leechdoms*, ed. Cockayne I, 121. [8] *Herbarium*, ed. de Vriend, pp. 128–9.
[9] *Ibid.*, pp. 244–5.
[10] *Ibid.*, pp. 40–1 and 288.

Cotton Vitellius C. iii seems for that reason to have omitted it altogether from his copy.[11]

Sometimes we cannot be sure that the error was the translator's fault. In ch. 4 of *MDQ* he translated *locis inferioribus* ('lower parts'), euphemistic for *womb, genitals*, by *inwerdlicum stowum* ('internal parts'), but maybe his exemplar had *interioribus* by mistake.[12] The same doubt applies to a recipe where he seems to have got two regions of the body confused. Ch. 5.5 of the *Herbarium* begins: *Ad pectinem mulierum* ('for women's pubes'). The Old English translation reads: *Gif wifes breost sare sien* ('if a woman's breasts are sore'). He appears to have confused *pecten* and *pectus*, but again the mistake may have already been in his exemplar.[13]

He also had trouble with measurements. For example, in ch. 10.1 he translated *scorpionis parte prima* ('in the early part of the sign of the Scorpion', i.e., in late October) as *on Octobre foreweardum* ('in early October').[14] (Or is this an indication that the Julian calendar was already out of phase with the seasons?) It is doubtful that he had any idea of the capacity of a *congius* (about 3.5 litres); in one place (36.3) he equated it with an *ambur* (about 27 litres), in another (41.1) with a *sester* (about 0.6 litre).[15] The tremissis he equated with various weights ranging from half a dragma to six dragmas; the penny with weights ranging from one-third scrupule to one dragma.[16] Obviously, he had only the vaguest notions of Mediterranean weights and measures.

He had no trouble with the animals in *MDQ*; they were the same ones he knew in England. But when it came to dealing with the plants of the *Herbarium* it was a different matter; these were from a Mediterranean flora and he was often at a loss to identify them, sometimes giving up and leaving the place for the English equivalent name blank in his text. In fact, he did not attempt an English translation for forty-one of the 185 plants in the complete *Herbarium*. Some of them are still doubtfully identifiable, but some of his omissions are surprising, such as *nymphea* (ch. 69: *nymphete*),[17] for which glosses elsewhere give the equivalent *colloncroh* ('water lily'), and for which in the manuscript there is a good illustration of a water lily. Even where he gave English names, these were frequently loanwords from his source. For further discussion, one should consult the

[11] *Ibid.*, pp. 242–3 and 268–9. [12] *Ibid.*, pp. 244–5. [13] *Ibid.*, pp. 50–1.
[14] *Ibid.*, pp. 54–5. [15] *Ibid.*, pp. 82–3 and 86–7.
[16] *Ibid.*, pp. lxxxii–lxxxiii.
[17] *Ibid.*, p. 110.

excellent analyses of plant-naming in the *Herbarium* carried out by M. A. D'Aronco.[18]

In spite of the Latin *Herbarium* being a collection of remedies using plants native to Mediterranean regions, there can be no doubt that the Anglo-Saxons found it useful, important enough to justify at least four copies in translation besides the Latin copies in their hands. The translation was not slavishly made; Linda Voigts has shown how the material of the individual chapters was re-arranged for greater ease of use. For example, the description of habitat, which in the Latin original usually came at the end of the chapter, was placed at the beginning. Invocations of plants, common in the Latin version, were almost all omitted from the translation. Voigts has also shown that surviving copies of the translation were supplied with a preliminary table detailing the contents of each chapter, and that in at least one copy (Cotton Vitellius C. iii), the rubricated initials of the table and chapters were coordinated.[19] There can be no doubt that these copies were not mindless scribal exercises but were made to be used.

PERI DIDAXEON

Peri Didaxeon[20] is of so late a date (late twelfth century) that it cannot be considered as an Anglo-Saxon treatise; even the language is doubtfully Old English, many commentators considering it as transitional between Old and Middle English. As we have it, it is incomplete, the last part of the manuscript being lost (or never completed by the translator). Löweneck has shown that much of it is a selective translation of material taken from *Petrocellus*; because Löweneck had only the first part of this work as edited by De Renzi, he was not able to show the full extent of the borrowing. Some chapters are not borrowed from *Petrocellus* (at least, as we have that work now); Löweneck shows no sources for these. The most that can be said about this vernacular version is that it shows that *Petrocellus* was popular in the twelfth century and that medical texts were still being written in English a century after the Conquest.

[18] M. A. D'Aronco, 'Inglese antico *galluc*', pp. 1–18; see also M. A. D'Aronco, 'The Botanical Lexicon of the OE "Herbarium"', *ASE* 17 (1988), 15–33.

[19] L. E. Voigts, 'Anglo-Saxon Plant Remedies and the Anglo-Saxons', *Isis* 70 (1979), 250–68.

[20] *Leechdoms*, ed. Cockayne III, 82–144; Löweneck, 'Peri Didaxeon', pp. 1–57.

9

Sources for Old English texts

In the preceding chapters I have frequently referred to borrowing by the Anglo-Saxons and to the knowledge of medicine they acquired from Mediterranean sources. It is time now to describe these sources and their availability to the Anglo-Saxons.

Until quite recently it was a common opinion that medieval medicine was rather poor stuff and that a medicine worthy of the name was introduced into Northern Europe only as a result of the impetus to learning supplied by the Arabs and introduced into Italy at Salerno when Constantinus Africanus began to teach there shortly before AD 1100. A careful analysis of the texts left to us from Anglo-Saxon England will show whether this opinion was justified. The best way to do this is to examine the sources of these texts and to compare them with their Greek, Roman, Byzantine, North African and native origins.

Because *Leechbook III* is the only representative of the corpus of ancient northern medicine surviving from the Anglo-Saxon period, our comparison of sources must be chiefly to the medicine of Mediterranean cultures. By comparing texts of Anglo-Saxon origin with contemporary and earlier Latin medical texts we can determine to some extent what medical texts of Mediterranean origin were known to the Anglo-Saxons and what use was made of them. Only works in Latin need to be considered, for there is no evidence that Anglo-Saxons other than those under the immediate teaching or influence of Theodore and Hadrian at Canterbury could handle Greek well enough to be able to use medical texts in Greek. However, most of the important post-Hippocratic medical works in Greek had been translated into Latin by the sixth and seventh centuries, or their substance transmitted in the form of epitomes or by incorporation into Latin collections.

To appreciate the use made of this Latin corpus, we must now examine it in some detail. Although Hippocrates and Galen were authorities to whom all writers paid lip service, very few of the authentic writings of either were available in the West in either Greek or Latin during the Anglo-Saxon period. Much of their teachings and practices, on the other hand, was available at second hand in quotations, summaries and reworkings in the compilations of later authors, often without acknowledgement and often in a debased form. On the other hand, when a medieval Latin text is assigned to Hippocrates or Galen, the attribution is almost always wrong, being merely an attempt by some author or scribe to lend authority to his material. After Galen, the most influential Greek writer to whom lip service was paid was Dioscorides, who had flourished in the first half of the first century AD, he and Pliny, the Roman encyclopaedist, being contemporaries. His *Materia medica*, an account of plants, animals and mineral products of medical value, was still actively used as late as the seventeenth century, and although it was translated into Latin early, its size restricted its use, as appears from the few copies which survive.[1] But if not used directly, it was edited and epitomized and various versions of these derived works survive usually under Dioscorides's name or that of Apuleius and often profusely illustrated. The illustrations became more and more stylized and unnatural with repeated copyings, but are in a line of plant and animal illustration going back to the earliest examples of naturalistic Greek illustration, antedating Dioscorides himself by centuries.

In the second century Philumenus, a younger contemporary of Galen and a member of the Eclectic School of medicine, wrote treatises on various subjects, most of which are lost. Some of his work on abdominal diseases survives in the *Practica Alexandri*, and in shorter extracts in the works of Oribasius.[2] Philagrius of Epirus flourished in Thessalonica in the fourth century and was an authority on diseases of the spleen.[3] Fragments of his work survive also in the *Practica Alexandri* and in the works of Oribasius.

---

[1] *Dioscuridis de Materia Medica*, ed. Wellmann. Greek manuscripts of Dioscorides were profusely illustrated, the most notable being the Juliana Anicia Codex of the sixth century (Vienna, Österreichische Nationalbibliothek, Vindobonensis Med. Gr. I). Copies of these illustrations are in *The Greek Herbal of Dioscorides, Illustrated by a Byzantine A.D. 512, Englished by J. Goodyear A.D. 1655; edited and first printed A.D. 1933 by R. T. Gunther* (Oxford, 1934).

[2] *Nachträge*, ed. Puschmann, is a convenient text for reference to the surviving works of Philumenus and Philagrius of Epirus. On the *Practica Alexandri*, see above, p. 22, n. 11. For Oribasius, see below, n. 4.

[3] See above, n. 2.

Oribasius, a native of Pergamon, where he received his medical training, was one of the three authors most influential in the transmission to later times of classical medicine in the tradition of Galen, the others being Cassius Felix of Numidia and Alexander of Tralles. Oribasius became physician to the emperor Julian, whom he accompanied on his Gaulish campaigns (355–60). It was while on these campaigns that he compiled his *Medical Collection* (Ἰατρικαὶ Συναγωγαὶ) in seventy books. In this massive encyclopaedia he cited at least thirty-one authorities by name. Near the end of his life, about 390, at the request of his son, who was also a physician, he reduced his encyclopaedia to convenient working dimensions in the nine books of the *Synopsis* (Σύνοψις), a handbook for trained physicians working in rural areas away from urban facilities. Still later, at the request of his biographer, who was a layman, he wrote the *Euporistes* (Εὐπόριστα), in four books, a manual of hygiene, simple medicines and descriptions of diseases for the use of laymen and having a relatively simple pharmacopoeia. In both these shorter works he borrowed freely from Galen and many other predecessors. Both the *Synopsis* and *Euporistes* were translated into Latin in the late sixth or early seventh century, not once but twice, so that it is a nice exercise to determine from which translation a later writer has borrowed.[4]

Vindicianus, friend and personal physician to St Augustine of Hippo, flourished about 364–75. He wrote on various subjects, chiefly gynaecology. His surviving fragments, collected by Rose, include parts of his gynaecological works, fragments of a more general work, the *Epitome altera*, and an *Epistula Vindiciani ad Pentadium nepotem*, which, as we have seen, was known to Bede and had a wide circulation in the Middle Ages.[5]

---

4 The Greek text and the complete Latin translations of Oribasius are in *Œuvres d'Oribase*, ed. U. C. Bussemaker and C. Daremberg, 6 vols. (Paris, 1856–76). Vols. V and VI contain the Greek texts of the *Synopsis* and *Euporistes*, together with the 'old' and 'new' Latin translations. Vol. VI was edited by A. Molinier after the two earlier editors had died; it contains an excellent account of the life, works and manuscript tradition of Oribasius. The most recent edition of the Greek Oribasius is *Oribasii Collectionum Medicarum Reliquiae*, ed. J. Raeder, 3 vols. (Berlin, 1928). On the dating of the 'old' and 'new' translations, see H. Mørland, *Die lateinischen Oribasiusübersetzungen* and *Oribasius Latinus (Erster Teil)*. Of the *Synopsis* and *Euporistes* some half-dozen manuscripts survive from our period; see Beccaria, *Codici*, p. 475. None is of English origin, but see J. D. A. Ogilvy, *Books Known to the English, 597–1066* (Cambridge, MA, 1967), p. 208, for a twelfth-century Oribasius manuscript containing English glosses.

5 See above, p. 28, n. 17.

Theodorus Priscianus was a disciple of Vindicianus and physician to the emperor Gratian (367–93). Only parts of his works survive together with a large collection of pseudo-Theodoran material attached to them. This collection also seems to have been widely known in the Middle Ages.[6]

Probably as early as the fourth century and certainly not later than the sixth, the work known as *Herbarium Apulei Platonici traditum a Chirone Centauro, magistro Achillis*, usually shortened to *Herbarium Apulei*, was compiled. This *Herbarium* attracted to itself other similar works; the extent of these has been described in the preceding chapter. Judging from the number of surviving manuscripts, this expanded *Herbarium* complex was very popular in the Middle Ages.[7]

Around the end of the fourth century, Marcellus of Bordeaux, sometimes labelled Empiricus, compiled a large collection of medical remedies, the *De medicamentis*, in thirty-six books.[8] He was not a physician and his recipes include, besides rational medical ones, many folk remedies and charms (some of them of Celtic, i.e., Gaulish, origin). The medical value of the work is low, but it is nevertheless of great interest to the student of medicine, because of the wide range of recipes it contains and because it was plundered freely in the Middle Ages. The few surviving manuscripts also contain epistles attributed to Hippocrates, Pliny and Celsus.

Caelius Aurelianus, a fifth-century physician of Sicca in Numidia, derived his massive text books, *Celeres vel acutae passiones* and *Tardae passiones*,[9] mostly from the works of Soranus of Ephesus, who flourished in the second century, but whose writings on general medicine and on gynaecology are largely lost. The books of Caelius were, like the encyclopaedia of Oribasius, too cumbersome for practical use and were epitomized, the epitomes themselves apparently being worked over to produce the *Liber Aurelii de acutis passionibus* and *Liber Esculapii de chronicis passionibus*, anonymous works having a wide circulation in the Middle Ages.

[6] *Ibid.*   [7] *Herbarium*, ed. de Vriend, Introduction, *passim*.

[8] *Marcelli De Medicamentis*, ed. Niedermann.

[9] The *Acutae passiones* and *Tardae passiones* survive only in printed editions. A good account of the works of Soranus and Caelius Aurelianus is in the introduction to *Caelius Aurelianus, On Acute Diseases and On Chronic Diseases*, ed. I. E. Drabkin (Chicago, 1950), where the *Aurelius* and *Esculapius* are also discussed. The *Aurelius* and *Esculapius* seem to have had no direct influence on Old English texts; that they were known in England is attested by their appearance in the manuscript Cambridge, Peterhouse, 251.

There also survive portions of a medical catechism believed to be a genuine work of Caelius. [10]

Cassius Felix, a physician of the Logical School who lived in Cirta, Numidia, wrote his little book, the *De medicina ex Graecis Logicae Sectae auctoribus liber translatus*, in 447. [11] It was his habit to give the original Greek terms alongside their Latin equivalents, for example, 'collectiones Graeci apostomata vocant'. This made his book a mine of material from which glossators and others dug out many of the Greek medical terms still used in Western medicine. His book was used by Isidore of Seville, and we have seen Bede quoting from it.

Alexander, who was born at Tralles in Lydia, Asia Minor (now Turkey) in 525, died at Rome in 605, having travelled extensively in his early years. He was a member of a talented Byzantine family and author of a treatise on fevers, and of another work in the head-to-foot tradition in twelve books, which survive, and of other shorter works which do not, although it is thought that short treatises on the eye attributed to him may actually be his. His major work was soon translated into Latin and augmented with material from Philumenus and Philagrius; these additions were apparently intended to supplement Alexander's work by treating subjects he had not discussed or had treated lightly. This *Practica Alexandri* was known throughout the Middle Ages. [12]

Universally known were the works of two encyclopaedists, the *Historia naturalis* of Pliny the Elder[13] and the *Etymologiae sive origines* of Isidore of Seville. [14] The medical parts of Pliny's work were often extracted and promulgated as separate works, sometimes arranged alphabetically or according to diseases or parts of the body, as in the *Medicina Plinii* and *Physica Plinii*. [15] Similarly, the fourth and eleventh

---

[10] *Anecdota Graeca*, ed. Rose II, 163–240.   [11] See above, p. 28, n. 18.

[12] *Alexander von Tralles*, ed. Puschmann. The short treatises on the eye are in *Nachträge*, ed. Puschmann. Some six manuscripts of the Latin version of Alexander survive from our period (Beccaria, *Codici*, p. 439); the *Practica* is also available in sixteenth-century editions; see above, p. 22, n. 11.

[13] The standard edition is *Plinii Naturalis Historiae Libri XXXVII*, ed. Mayhoff and Jan; Pliny, *HN* VI–VIII; see above, p. 37, n. 6.

[14] *Isidori Hispalensis Episcopi Etymologiarum sive Originum, Libri XX*, ed. W. M. Lindsay, 2 vols. (Oxford, 1911). Bk IV ('De medicina'), bk XI ('De homine et portentis') and bk XVII ('De rebus rusticis') are of most interest to students of medical history.

[15] The medieval reworking of Pliny's medical material has been edited as *Medicina Plinii*, ed. Önnerfors; see above, p. 37, n. 6.

books of Isidore's *Etymologiae* sometimes formed independent works.[16]

There is a large amount of scattered recipe material and of short treatises on various aspects of medicine, still mostly unedited and unprinted, much of it from the period we are dealing with here. There are tractates on bloodletting, accounts of the four humours, prognostics of life and death, dietaries and so on, some published, many still in manuscript, and usually anonymous or attributed to one or another famous person of the past, even Plato and Alexander the Great.

One group of texts must be given special mention. In 1854, Salvatore De Renzi published from a twelfth-century manuscript (Paris, Bibliothèque Nationale, lat. 24025) a work which he entitled the *Practica Petrocelli Salernitani*, Petrocellus being an eleventh-century Salernitan writer.[17] But the attribution is incorrect, because copies of the work survive from as early as the late ninth century. Moreover, De Renzi did not edit the whole of the work; in the Sloane and Harley collections of the British Library,[18] for example, there are copies of the work which include a second book, of which De Renzi gave only a chapter list and the content of a couple of chapters. This second part remains unpublished. For want of a better title we may continue to call the whole work the *Practica Petrocelli*, or simply *Petrocellus*, although it seems to have sometimes gone by the title of its opening epistle, given variously in the manuscripts as *Peri Didaxeon* or *Peri Hereseon*. Another work in the same class is the *Passionarius Galeni*, containing much material at second or third hand from the works of Galen and attributed to the Salernitan writer Gariopontus since the twelfth century at least. There is good reason to suppose that Gariopontus's contribution was to edit and correct an existing work and that this has led to the attribution of the authorship to him.[19]

[16] W. D. Sharpe, 'Isidore of Seville: the Medical Writings. An English Translation with an Introduction and Commentary', *Transactions of the American Philosophical Society* ns 54 (1964), 1–75, has an excellent commentary to bks IV and XI.

[17] *Collectio Salernitana*, ed. De Renzi; the *Practica Petrocelli Salernitani* is at IV, 185–291.

[18] Both parts of the *Petrocellus* are in London, BL, Sloane 2839; there is also a copy (the second part being incomplete) in London, BL, Harley 4977.

[19] Apart from manuscript copies, there are at least two printed editions of the *Passionarius Galeni* from the sixteenth century, attributed to Gariopontus: *Passionarius Galeni* and *Garioponti ad totius corporis aegritudines remediorum . . . libri V . . . de febribus . . . libri II*, etc. (Basel, 1531). De Renzi, discussing Gariopontus (*Collectio Salernitana* I, 137–49), quotes from a Basel manuscript (not further identified): 'Passionarium, seu practica morborum Galieni, Theodori Prisciani, Alexandri et Pauli, quem Gariopontus quidam

Neither the *Petrocellus* nor the *Passionarius* is an original work. Both are compiled from earlier medical works. This is particularly true of the *Passionarius*, which, in spite of its title, seems to quote directly from almost everyone except Galen. The *Petrocellus* leans heavily on Cassius Felix, often beginning a chapter with a quotation from his book and sometimes quoting a whole chapter from it as a whole chapter of the *Petrocellus*. It also shares much material with the *Passionarius*, both having drawn on the same sources, and to some extent it borrows from Alexander and from other early collections such as the *Liber teropetici*, which survives in only a couple of manuscripts.[20] When we come to examine Bald's *Leechbook* in detail, we will be struck by the similar arrangements of the two works, which leads me to suspect that the *Petrocellus* may be the product of an English compiler. I have not made a sufficiently close study of the work to be more specific about its origins.

To appreciate the position of these two collections in medieval medicine, we must look at a group of shorter treatises whose composition seems to be not later than the seventh or early eighth century. Two of them have already been mentioned, the *Liber Aurelii* and the *Liber Esculapii*, both derived from the works of Caelius Aurelianus. Often accompanying them in manuscripts are four short treatises purporting to be the work of Galen. These are *Galeni ad Glauconem de medendi methodo Liber I*, *Galeni ad Glauconem de mendendi methodo Liber II*, *Galeni Liber tertius* and *Galeni de podagra*.[21] Galen did address short works to his friend Glaucon, but these little treatises, while sharing to some extent the same subject material and following Galenic precepts, are in no sense translations of those which Galen wrote for Glaucon. But they form a large part of the *Passionarius*, which is made up in general by taking a chapter on a given subject from *Aurelius* or *Esculapius* and following that by a second and even a third

Salernitanus, eiusque Socii, una cum Albicio emendavit, ab erroribus vindicavit et in hunc ordinem redegit' (*'Passionarius*, or *Practice of Disease* of Galen, Theodorus Priscianus, Alexander and Paulus, which Gariopontus, a certain Salernitan, and his associates, together with Albicius, corrected, cleared of errors and arranged in this order'). This implies editing, not composing.

[20] London, BL, Arundel 166 (12r–90v); Paris, Bibliothèque Nationale, lat. 11219 (118v), both of the ninth century.

[21] These six treatises were all available to Anglo-Saxons; for example, the manuscript Cambridge, Peterhouse 251 (St Augustine's, Canterbury, s. xi[ex]) contains texts of all of them. See H. Gneuss, 'A Preliminary List of Manuscripts Written or Owned in England up to 1100', *ASE* 9 (1981), 1–60, at 13 (no. 145).

chapter on the same subject from *Liber I*, *Liber II* or *Liber tertius*. Bk IV of the *Passionarius* (on gout) is virtually a direct copy of the *Galeni de podagra*, so that when *Petrocellus* seems to have borrowed from the *Passionarius* (or vice versa) the borrowing may in fact have been from these other works. The result of this free borrowing is that, when one is looking for source texts, one is often in a quandary as to which of these interrelated works was in the borrower's hands. This will become obvious when we look at the making of Bald's *Leechbook*.

Two works attributed (no doubt, falsely) to Soranus of Ephesus seem to have been used by the Anglo-Saxons. The *Quaestiones medicinales* are known from only two manuscripts,[22] and are without doubt the source of the glosses to one of the two little medical poems in the *Canterbury Classbook* manuscript (discussed above, p. 49). The other little set of verses (a list of forty-seven medical terms, most of them Greek) owes much to a medical glossary printed in Goetz's *Corpus Glossariorum Latinorum* from two manuscripts (one of the tenth, the other of the early eleventh century).[23] An interesting collection, the *Sorani Ephesii Vetustissimi Archiatri et Peripatetici, in Artis Medendi Isagogen*, was edited by A. Thorin at Basel in 1528. No manuscript of this collection is known; it contains material from the *Quaestiones medicinales*, and the usual assembly of short tracts on diet, bloodletting, humours, etc., found in medieval medical manuscripts. Much of its contents is also found in the *Liber teropetice* in a section of that work entitled *De arte prolixa*;[24] neither work can claim to be the source of the other. Many of its contents appear also in the Latin collections made by the Anglo-Saxons.

Very rarely is a source mentioned in the leechbooks, but there is one named source of special interest. In Bald's *Leechbook* there is a chapter for which the headnote reads:

A medicine: scammony for constipation of the inwards and 'gutamon' for pain in the spleen and stitch, and spikenard (?) for diarrhoea, and tragacanth for corrupt phlegms in men, and aloes for infirmities, and galbanum for shortness of breath,

22 London, BL, Cotton Galba E. iv, of the thirteenth century, and Chartres, Bibliothèque Municipale, 62, of the late tenth (this manuscript was destroyed in the 1939–45 war). The Cotton *QM* was published in *Anecdota Graeca*, ed. Rose II, 243–74, and part of the Chartres *QM* by Stadler, 'Neue Bruchstücke', pp. 361–8.

23 *Corpus Glossariorum Latinorum*, ed. G. Goetz, 7 vols. (Leipzig, 1888–1923) III, 596–607, from Vatican City, Biblioteca Apostolica Vaticana, Reg. lat. 1260, 177v–178r, and Bern, Burgerbibliothek, 337, 8r–14v.

24 London, BL, Arundel 166, 82v–86v.

and balsam anointing for all infirmities, and petroleum to drink alone for inward tenderness and to smear on outwardly, and theriac is a good drink for inward tenderness, and the white stone for all unknown afflictions.[25]

Unfortunately, the opening part of the chapter is lost with the lost leaves of the manuscript, the existing text starting in the middle of the uses for balsam. It is the closing sentence which gives the chapter its unusual interest: 'All this Domnus Elias, patriarch of Jerusalem, ordered to be said to King Alfred.'[26] According to Asser, Alfred's biographer, Elias sent letters and gifts to Alfred; from Asser and from Alfred himself we also learn that Alfred suffered from some distressing but undiagnosed ailment. It is likely that among the letters and gifts from the patriarch were medicines and directions for their use, so that in this chapter we have a clue to the exchange of goods and ideas between England and the Near East and to the date at which the *Leechbook* may have been compiled, which, according to this chapter, could not be earlier than the later years of Alfred's reign.

[25] *Leechdoms*, ed. Cockayne II, 174; 'Læcedom se monian [*read* scamonian] wiþ innoþes forhæfdnesse 7 gutomon, wið milte wærce 7 stice 7 spican wiþ utsihtan 7 dracontian wiþ fule horas on men, 7 alwan wiþ untrymnessum, 7 galbanes wiþ nearwum breostum, 7 balzaman smiring wiþ eallum untrumnessum 7 petraoleum to drincanne anfeald wiþ innan tydernesse 7 utan to smerwanne, 7 tyriaca is god drenc wiþ innoþ tydernessum, 7 se hwita stan wið eallum uncuþum brocum.' The remains of the chapter are on pp. 288–90.

[26] *Ibid.*, p. 290. 'þis eal het þus secgean ælfrede cyninge domne helias patriarcha on gerusalem.'

10

Making a *Leechbook*

There is nothing new under the sun, nor can anyone say: Behold, this is new: for already it was in the old times which were before us. [1]

The survival from periods not too far apart of three more or less complete medical works compiled in Old English – Bald's *Leechbook*, *Leechbook III* and the *Lacnunga* – gives an excellent opportunity to examine how such compilations were made, to find their sources and to see how those sources were used and so to give an insight into the understanding and practice of medicine by the Anglo-Saxons.

It was never the intention of an ancient or medieval medical writer to be wholly original, but rather to reproduce authoritative materials from the past. When an Anglo-Saxon physician or scribe set out to compile a medical collection, he might have had as many as three sources to call upon: Latin works or their translations incorporating the medical lore of Greek, Roman, North African and Byzantine cultures; native northern medicines already in medical compilations; traditional or new remedies never before written down. It is both interesting and instructive to try to trace entries in the surviving Old English texts to these sources, although the attempt can be beset with formidable difficulties. In the first place, because the surviving vernacular medical texts of Anglo-Saxon England are the oldest in Northern Europe, we have no anterior northern material with which to compare them. In the second place, although the amount of material surviving in Latin and Greek is very large, collections have been lost without trace. Consequently, when we cannot find a source or analogue

[1] Eccles. I.10: 'Nihil sub sole novum, nec valet quisquam dicere: Ecce hoc recens est: iam enim præcessit in sæculis, quæ fuerunt ante nos.'

for an entry in an Anglo-Saxon work we can only guess at its origin. Even when we have analogous remedies from earlier works, we cannot always be sure that the Anglo-Saxon compiler drew from these works directly or got his material at second or third hand through intermediaries which may or may not still exist, or even that he may have been using common folk medicines of northern and Mediterranean cultures not yet reduced to writing.

These problems will become more intelligible if we examine Old English remedies and their probable sources and analogues in more detail than was done in ch. 6. There is reason to think that *Leechbook III* comes closest to being a collection of native medicines, its background being mostly in the northern traditions for which sources do not exist, it itself being the oldest survivor of its kind. As we saw in ch. 6, most of its analogues with the Latin tradition are found in the *Herbarium* and in *Marcellus*, amounting to less than one third of the total number of entries. A few examples will suffice to show these relationships. 'If there is a bone broken in the head and it will not come away, pound green betony and lay on the wound frequently until the bones come away and the wound is better.'[2] The *Herbarium* version reads: 'For a fracture of the head. The herb betony pounded and laid on the blow on the head closes up the wound and heals it wonderfully quickly.'[3] These treatments are in the same tradition and for the same condition but the one in the *Leechbook* is concerned with ridding the wound of splinters of bone and the one in the *Herbarium* with proper closure of the wound. Again: 'For an ulcerated mouth take plum-tree leaves, boil in wine and wash out the mouth with it.'[4] A similar one in *Marcellus* reads: 'Plum-tree leaves are cooked in wine; their expressed juice held in the mouth is very good.'[5] This was a widespread treatment given also by Dioscorides, Pliny, Gargilius and in two other places by Marcellus, as well as being in the *Physica Plinii*. Given such wide distribution, it is difficult to claim that this remedy was borrowed from any one of these authorities rather than that it belonged to a common

[2] *Leechdoms*, ed. Cockayne II, 326–8: 'Gif gebrocen ban sie on heafde 7 of nelle, cnua grene betonican 7 lege on þæt dolh gelome oþ þæt þa ban of syn 7 þæt dolh gebatod.'

[3] *Herbarium*, ed. de Vriend, p. 31: 'Ad capitis fracturam. Herba vettonica contusa et super capitis ictu imposita vulnus mira celeritate glutinatum sanabit.'

[4] *Leechdoms*, ed. Cockayne II, 310: 'Wiþ innan tobrocenum muðe nim plum treowes leaf, wyl on wine 7 swile mid þone muþ.'

[5] *Marcelli De Medicamentis*, ed. Niedermann, p. 204: 'Arboris pruni folia cum uino decoquuntur; eorum sucus expressus intra os retentus plurimum prodest.'

background of European traditional medicine. This one also appears to belong to a common tradition: 'If sinews are cut through, take earthworms, pound well, lay on until they are healed.'[6] Dioscorides wrote: 'Earthworms pounded and laid on conglutinate severed sinews'.[7] A similar recipe is found in *Marcellus* and in *Theodorus Priscianus*, but with more complicated preparations and with added ingredients. Even the old Latin translation of Dioscorides adds to the original: 'Earthworms *which are found in dung*, pounded and laid on conglutinate severed sinews'.[8] Although it is extremely doubtful that the compiler of *Leechbook III* was acquainted with Dioscorides's *Materia medica*, his form of the recipe is closest to the Greek one; the simplest explanation is that both were taken from a common oral source.

Other recipes are clearly borrowed from the Latin literature. An example is: 'For strained-out bile eat radish and pepper after the night's fast and with it sup linseed boiled in milk, do this frequently, he will soon be well.'[9] Marcellus gave the same recipe: 'To restrain bile: If anyone eats fasting radish with pepper and linseed it will strongly inhibit strained-out bile.'[10] 'Strained-out bile' is found also in another remedy in *Leechbook III* and is also in *Lacnunga* and appears to be of Latin origin, so we may conclude that its presence in a recipe indicates that the Old English depends directly or indirectly on a Latin one. This one also must have been borrowed: 'For pain in the stomach, rue seed and quicksilver and vinegar, eat after the night's fast.'[11] The *Herbarium* reads: 'For pain in the stomach. Seed of the herb rue with live sulphur and vinegar taste fasting.'[12] It is

---

[6] *Leechdoms*, ed. Cockayne II, 328: 'Gif sinwe syn forcorfene nim renwyrmas, gecnuwa wel, lege on oþ þæt hi hale synd.'

[7] *Dioscuridis Materia Medica*, ed. Wellmann I, 142: γῆς ἔντερα λεῖα ἐπιτεθέντα νεύρων διακοπὰς κολλᾷ ('Earthworms ground up and laid on conglutinate severed sinews').

[8] *Dioscorides Longobardus*, ed. H. Stadler, *Romanische Forschungen* 10 (1895), 181–247, at 195: '(Gisentera) quae in stercore inuenitur, trita et inposita neruorum concisiones coagulat'.

[9] *Leechdoms*, ed. Cockayne II, 314: 'Wiþ seondum geallan ete rædic 7 pipor on neahtnestig 7 awylled linsæd on meolce supe mid, do þus gelome, him biþ sona sel.'

[10] *Marcelli De Medicamentis*, ed. Niedermann, p. 534: 'Ad bilem reprimendam: Rafanum ex pipere et lini semine si quis ieiunus manducauerit, fortissime bilem expressam inhibebit.'

[11] *Leechdoms*, ed. Cockayne II, 356: 'Wiþ magan wærce, rudan sæd 7 cwicseolfor 7 eced bergen on neahtnestig.'

[12] *Herbarium*, ed. de Vriend, p. 135: 'Ad stomachi dolorem. Herbae rutae semen cum sulfure vivo et aceto ieiunus gustato.'

doubtful that 'live sulphur' could have been transformed into quicksilver (mercury) except through mistaken translation from Latin.

Most of the remedies in *Leechbook III* are not found in the medical literature in Latin and may be presumed to be of native origin, and some of those which have analogues in the Latin literature are sufficiently different to indicate that they may not have been borrowed and can be presumed to be of native origin. The implication is that much of *Leechbook III* represents a native northern element of Anglo-Saxon medicine.

Bald's *Leechbook* is quite a different thing. Its outstanding characteristic is its integration of native medicine with an extensive and selective borrowing from the Latin literature. Moreover, it differs from the standard medical compendium in that bk I deals with external or externally manifested conditions, whereas bk II deals with internal ones, as its first sentence makes clear:[13] 'These treatments apply to all internal infirmities.' These two characteristics make it unique among medieval collections. To appreciate the compiler's technique and his use of sources, we may examine a fairly long extract and compare it in detail with its sources and analogues. In it I have numbered items of the original and their sources/analogues to facilitate comparisons.[14]

[1] If you wish for your belly to be always healthy, then if you will, you should treat it thus: Every day see that your faeces and urine be healthy as is right. If the urine is scanty cook celery and fennel, make a good broth or juice and of other sweet herbs. If the faeces are too few, take the herb which in the south is called turpentine, as much as an oil berry (i.e., olive); give it when he wishes to go to bed. These herbs are also very good for that and easier to get: beet and mallow and cabbage and the likes of these, cooked together with the flesh of young swine; let him take the broth, and also nettle cooked in water and salted is to be eaten, and also elder leaves and the broth in the same way. Some give aloe leaves when one is about to go to bed, as much as three beans every day to be swallowed, and drinks like these, and stronger ones, if need be, are to be given, especially in early spring before the harmful humour, which had collected in winter, is diffused through the other limbs. Many people have not heeded this, nor heed it [now]; then there results from the harmful humours either hemiplegia or falling sickness or the white scurf (which in the south is called leprosy), or tetter or scurf on the head or erysipelas. Therefore the harmful humours must

[13] *Leechdoms*, ed. Cockayne II, 158: 'Þas læcedomas belimpað to eallum innoþa mettrymnessum.'

[14] *Leechdoms*, ed. Cockayne II, 164, for the headnote; *ibid.* 226–30 for the main text: see Appendix 1 (below, pp. 187–8) for the Old English texts.

first be cleansed away before the illnesses come and increase in the winter and spread through the limbs.

[2] For disease and pain of the belly: Linseed rubbed or beaten, a bowl full, and two of sharp vinegar, boil down together, give to the sick one to drink after the night's fast. Again: Lay chewed pennyroyal on the navel, it will be calmed at once. Again: Rub in water a little dill seed, give to drink. For disease of the belly and for pain of the bowels: When the belly is disordered because of much chill do those things which we wrote about above. Then if the belly be upset or irritated, take three bunches of laurel shoots, rub, and single spoonfuls of cumin and parsley and twenty peppercorns, rub all together and dry three membranes from young birds' bellies, after that take water, rub dill into it, and heat these things, give to drink until the pain is relieved.

[3] For the same: Take bread, boil in goat's milk, soak in southern drink. For belly disease: Boil rue in oil and let eat in oil. Again: A wild pigeon cooked in vinegar and in water, give to eat.

[4] For belly disease again: Let chew laurel leaves and swallow the juice and lay the leaves on the navel.

[5] Again: Hart's marrow melted, give to drink in hot water. For regulating the belly: Take beet, dig up and shake (do not wash it), but cook it for a long time in a kettle and boil it until it is all thoroughly cooked, and coagulated thick, then add a little salt and five spoonfuls of honey, oil one spoonful, give a bowlful.

[6] Again: A headed leek cooked, give a single one to eat. Again: Red nettle seed on bread, give to eat. Again: Mulberry juice, give to drink. Again: Plum shoots, eat after the night's fast. Again: Elder rind beaten, one pennyweight, give to drink a bowlful in cold water.

Item [1] of this long chapter may be compared with Oribasius's *Euporistes* I. 16. I give the whole of Oribasius's chapter, putting in italics those parts used by the *Leechbook* compiler so that we can see how he selected what he wanted for his own account. [15]

About those for whom it is useful that a healthy belly be always open. From the beginning it has always been the opinion of the ancients that for the sake of health the belly should be open every day, and a blameless emission of urine should take place following administration of food and drink. If these should not at all follow, then it is necessary to use those things which expel them and procure the compliance of the belly and urine. *If the supply of urine be less, decoctions are used in which are cooked chervil and smallage and fennel and asparagus; but if the belly is constipated, Chios turpentine the size of an olive is to be given to be swallowed when going to bed.* For those wishing more action a bit of

---

[15] *Œuvres d'Oribase*, ed. Molinier (*Euporistes*, I. 16); see Appendix 1 (below, pp. 188–9) for the Latin text.

natron is to be mixed in. *But more useful for moving the belly are potherbs, such as beet and mallow and cabbage cooked together, and a broth of the fresh flesh of swine.* But if these seem to be mild and one desires a stronger agent, then to provoke urine add parsley, carrot, anise, wormwood and grass and maidenhair fern and roots of edible thistle and medick and calamint and marjoram; each of them or with starch cooked in water, give to drink with wine; for all this purges the blood through the urine and is of no little help to the body. But if the things written here move the belly too gently and they desire to have more opening ones, *give salt cooked with herb mercury in water and when he has eaten it let him drink water; the leaves of elder similarly made up and taken work in this manner,* and the powder of fifty-two polypody roots made very fine on sardines and cooked in barley broth open the belly. *And some give when going to bed aloes as much as three chick pea seeds to swallow each day, and their belly is abundantly opened. Others also put thistle in broth so that it is cooked ground up together.* Of all these mentioned above it is better and more useful to drink epithymum in wine. But he who drinks it should have some supper, but less than usual and so pause; for it moves the belly slowly; but if he wishes to move it more, let him drink epithymum fasting in oximel. *But let him do this in early spring before the superabundant humour collected in winter boils up and is poured out and runs through some parts of the body and generates dangerous illnesses. For many who are careless suddenly fall into paralysis or apoplexy which these things cause, and others are seen to suffer ulcerations or similar scaly conditions, such as are leprosy or tetters, others scurf on the head, erysipelas and shingles. Therefore he is advised, so that some or none of this mischief may come, that he ought to purge before the humours collected in winter boil up, are dispersed and run through the body.*

It is instructive to speculate on why parts of this chapter were chosen and parts omitted. Some omitted parts, such as the first one, are merely comments on the success of a regimen of diet or medicine. Some remedies may have been omitted because the ingredients in them were not all easy to procure, such as the 'nitrum' to be added to a weaker medicine. For some omissions, it appears that the original may not have been understood; for example, one would normally take 'epitimus' to mean 'epitema' (επίθεμα), a cloth impregnated with a medicine and applied to the abdomen, whereas in Oribasius's text the 'epitimus' is to be drunk and so must be a potion made from epithymum, i.e., dodder (*Cuscuta epithymum*), which was used as a purge. These reasons suggested for omissions are only guesses on our part; the fact is that the compiler selected only parts of the chapter, choosing about half of it.

Item [2] of the Old English chapter (the next four remedies) comes from a series of six remedies in the *Physica Plinii* (there can be little doubt about

79

the source of these four remedies, as they are found in the same order in *Physica Plinii*):[16]

For pain or illness of the belly: (1) The dry powder of earth apple [*malum terre*] 6 scruples in 3 cups of wine given to drink, effectively relieves pain. (2) *Again: give to the fasting sufferer one-half pint of linseed bruised in one pint of strong vinegar and boiled thoroughly; it helps wonderfully.* (3) Again: the ashes of burned bread pounded with three cups of wine given to drink removes pain. (4) *Again: pennyroyal chewed and laid on the navel immediately removes pain.* (5) *Again for injuries of the belly: A little dill seed ground up in water is given to drink, immediately it corrects pain in the belly and cures the pain.* (6) *Again for injuries of the belly or all pains of the intestines: if the belly is costive from too much cold do as we have written above, but if there are cramps pound four laurel berries and a spoonful each of cumin and parsley, twenty pepper corns, pound up together and pound dry the membranes from the bellies of pullets, then drink with hot dilled water by potions until the pain is stilled.*

Recipes 1 and 3 were not copied; it is not clear just what plant was meant by 'malum terre'; three have been known by that name, birthwort (*Aristolochia rotunda*), species of *Cyclamen* and mandrake (*Mandragora officinarum*). According to a gloss quoted by Cockayne, mandrake was *eorðæppel* in Old English; if so, it would be unobtainable in England, as the plant is too tender to be successfully cultivated there. This may be why recipe 1 was not copied. I cannot think of a reason for the omission of recipe 3. Recipe 4 was a popular one; it is found also in the *Herbarium* and in *Leechbook III*.

The remedies of item [5] are found in the Latin *Herbarium* complex: the first of them in *Medicina de quadrupedibus*: 'For pain of the intestines and if there are cramps. Melted hart's marrow, give to drink in hot water, it heals wonderfully.'[17] The second one is found in the *Herbarium* chapter on *herba*

[16] *Physica Plinii*, ed. Önnerfors, p. 116; 'Ad uentris dolore uel uitia. (1) Malum terre siccum puluerem ∋ VI ex uino cyatos III potui datum dolorem efficaciter relebat. (2) *Item lini seminis cotila una in aceti acri cotilis duabus contusi et deferuefacti laboranti ieiuno dabis, mire iubabit.* (3) Item panis conbusti cinis tritus cum uini cyatis tribus potui datus dolorem tollit. (4) *Item puleium commanducatum et umbilico adpositum continuo dolore tollit.* (5) *Item ad uentris uitia: aneti seminis paululum tritum ex aqua potui datur, continuo dolorem uentris emendat, et dolore curebit.* (6) *Item ad uentris uitia uel omnes dolores interaneorum: siquidem nimio frigare uenter difficilis fuerit, facies ut superius scripsimus, si uero tortiones fuerint, iiii bacas lauri teris et cimini et petrisilini coclearia singula plena, piper grana xx simul conteris et teris pelliculis de uentribus pullorum sicca, exinde cum aqua anetata procallida bibat per potiones quam diu dolor sedatur.'*

[17] *Herbarium*, ed. de Vriend, p. 245: 'Ad intestinorum dolorem et si torminata fuerint, medulla ceruina remissa, potui dabis in aqua calida, mire sanat.'

prosepis (*gl.* 'id est personacia'): 'For pain in the intestines. Juice of the herb *personata*, let him drink fasting one cupful in two cupfuls of honey.'[18] 'Personata', 'personaca', 'personacia', 'prosepis' were all names for a plant which has been identified in the Latin literature with the greater burdock (*Arctium lappa*), but appears to have been taken by the Anglo-Saxons to be the beet. In herbal medicine burdock is recommended for intestinal troubles, beet is not. The *Leechbook* recipe using beet is more detailed than the *Herbarium* one, indicating that it was not borrowed at first hand.

The remaining remedies have most of their sources/analogues in the *Medicina Plinii*. Those of item [3] come from a single chapter: 'For cramps . . . bread cooked in goat's milk is taken twice a day in the form of a broth.'[19] This recipe well illustrates the changes which can happen in transmission through various languages over a long time. Dioscorides recommended millet roasted and put into a sack, placed warm on the abdomen for cramps.[20] Pliny recommended millet in this way: 'It checks loose bowels cooked in goat's milk and drunk twice a day.'[21] It is found in the same form in the *Medicina Plinii*,[22] but also in the recipe just quoted in which bread is found instead of millet. In this latter form it appears in *Marcellus*: 'Old bread cooked in goat's milk and given twice a day in the form of a broth to one suffering from loose bowels quickly helps.'[23] Apparently, the similarity of bread (*panis*) and millet (*panicum*) led to the change; it probably made little difference as neither millet nor bread is known to have much effect on the activity of the bowels, but it was in the bread version that it entered the Old English repertory.

The next two read: 'Rue is cooked in six cups of oil and the oil is drunk';

---

[18] *Ibid.*, p. 85: 'Ad intestinorum dolorem. Herbae personaciae sucus, cyatus i, ex melle cyatis duobus, ieiunus bibat.'

[19] *Medicina Plinii*, ed. Önnerfors, p. 43: 'Torminibus . . . panis cum lacte caprino decoctus bis in die sumitur more sorbitionis.'

[20] *Dioscuridis Materia Medica*, ed. Wellmann I, 174: [κέγχρος] φωχθεῖσα δὲ καὶ βληθεῖσα εἰς σάκκους πυριωμένη στρόφων καὶ τῶν ἄλλων ἀλγημάτων ἐστὶ βοήθημα '([millet] toasted and put hot into bags is good for gripings and other pains').

[21] Pliny, *HN* XXII.131: '[Panicum] . . . Sistit alvum in lacte caprino decoctum et bis die haustum.'

[22] *Medicina Plinii*, ed. Önnerfors, p. 41.

[23] *Marcellus*, ed. Niedermann, p. 478: 'Panis antiquus ex lacte caprino decoctus et more sorbitionis uentris fluxu laboranti bis ad diem datus cito succurret.'

'*A wild pigeon cooked in dilute vinegar is given as food.*'[24] According to Marcellus, the wild pigeon was to be cooked in raisin wine (*pusca*).

The remedies of part 6 are also all from the *Medicina Plinii*. The sources/analogues read: 'Headed leeks cooked up by themselves are taken in food.'[25] According to Marcellus, they should be eaten with vinegar.[26] 'For softening the belly . . . nettle seed toasted is collected with bread.'[27] One wonders if the 'red nettle' of the English recipe and the omission of 'toasted' point to differences in the text used from the ones we now have. Marcellus's version is essentially the same as that in the *Medicina Plinii*. The next two sources read: 'The juice of mulberries is given to drink';[28] 'The water in which wild plums are cooked is drunk.'[29] Pliny gave: 'Plums by themselves soften the belly.'[30] The next one is: 'One pennyweight of pounded elm bark in a hemina of cold water also purges.'[31] The substitution in the Old English recipe of 'elnes' ('of elder') for what should have been 'elmes' ('of elm') is most probably a scribe's error in copying from an earlier Old English translation, there being no similarity in Latin between *ulmus* ('elm') and *sambucus* ('elder'). This error shows that here the compiler of the *Leechbook* may have been taking his recipe from an English, not a Latin, collection, but again it may have been the fault of the scribe of our surviving manuscript. No source/analogue has been found for the remedy in part 4.

This long chapter with its analysis illustrates most of the techniques of composition used in Bald's *Leechbook*, showing that a typical chapter was made up from a selection of items taken from a number of works. These selections were assembled into a coherent whole, dealing with the subject given at the beginning of the chapter. One has the impression that an experienced physician was at work here, picking out what he had found

---

[24] *Medicina Plinii*, ed. Önnerfors, pp. 43 ('In oleo cyathis sex ruta decoquitur idque oleum bibitur') and 41 ('Palumbus ferus in cibo datur decoctus in pusca.').

[25] *Ibid.*, p. 40: 'Porri capitati discocti per se in cibo sumuntur.'

[26] *Marcellus*, ed. Niedermann, p. 368: 'Porri capitati excocti in cibo sumpti cum aceto plurimum prosunt stomacho laboranti.'

[27] *Medicina Plinii*, ed. Önnerfors, p. 40: 'Ventri molliendo . . . urticae semen *tostum* pane colligitur.'

[28] *Ibid.*, p. 40: 'Mororum maturorum sucus potui datur.'

[29] *Ibid.*, p. 41: 'Aqua in qua pruna agrestia cocta sint bibitur.'

[30] Pliny, *HN* XXIII.132: 'Ipsa pruna aluum molliunt.'

[31] *Medicina Plinii*, ed. Önnerfors, p. 40: 'Ulmi corticis tunsi denarii pondus in hemina aquae frigidae etiam purgat.'

useful in his practice and arranging it in a manner convenient for others to use, leaving out everything that he thought did not contribute to the subject of his chapter or which might confuse others less skilled than himself. Evidence of the care taken in composing the chapter is shown by the chapter-heading, which announces sixteen treatments and all sixteen appear in the text. (In contrast, recall the section of *Lacnunga* where twenty-eight remedies are announced and only thirteen given.) But evidence of careless revision also appears; the fourth remedy of part 2 ends with the words 'do ða þing to þe we be ufan writon', but in fact nothing pertinent was given above; the words were translated from the source text, where they did refer to an earlier treatment.

Large parts of Bald's *Leechbook* are made up in this way, not only from the sources given above, but also from the *Practica Alexandri*, the group of related texts making up the *Passionarius*, *Petrocellus*, and *Liber tertius*, as well as other shorter works, all used in the same fashion as in the example just given. This is particularly true of bk II, but there are also several instances in the more traditionally composed bk I. We have already discussed in ch. 6 the puzzling section on erysipelas, gangrene and amputation, with its unresolved problems of origin and arrangement. There is much that we do not know about the distribution of medical lore in Anglo-Saxon times.

When I first studied Bald's *Leechbook* and its sources, I assumed that a passage in the *Leechbook* which is virtually an exact translation of a Latin text implied direct borrowing by its compiler, but that deviations from such close agreement implied that the compiler took his material at second hand through an intermediate source. If this assumption were correct, we would have some idea of the contents of Bald's library, or what books were available to him. But recent work by A. L. Meaney has shown me the error of this assumption. It is worthwhile to give another fairly long quotation from the *Leechbook* to show how Meaney's evidence can tell us much about the state of medical literature in Bald's time. Here are the first nineteen remedies of ch. II of bk I, together with sources/analogues for most of them.[32]

1. 'Medicines for dimness of the eyes: take the juice or blossoms of celandine, mix with bumblebees' honey, put in a brass vessel, make lukewarm skilfully over warm coals until it is cooked. This is a good medicine for dimness of the eyes.'

[32] These nineteen remedies are found in *Leechdoms*, ed. Cockayne II, 26–30; for the Old English text see Appendix 1 (below, pp. 189–90).

Herbarium 75.2: 'For dimness of the eyes. Juice of the herb celandine or its flower expressed and mixed with Attic honey in a brass vessel, mixed together and cooked slowly over hot coals is a singular remedy for dimness of the eyes. Some use the juice alone.'[33]

Pliny, *HN* XXV.90: 'The juice of the flowering plants is expressed and is boiled down gently with Attic honey in a copper (brass) vessel over hot ashes, being a matchless remedy for dimness of the eyes.'[34]

2. 'For the same again: the juice of wild rue bedewed and brayed, mix with an equal amount of strained honey, anoint the eyes with that.'

Physica Plinii 17.27: 'Again: braying wild rue with its dew and its juice with strained honey, put equal weights and anoint; it benefits wonderfully.'[35]

3. 'For dimness of the eyes: Many people, in case their eyes should suffer from the complaint, look into cold water and then can see far; nor does it harm the sight, but much drinking of wine and other sweet drinks and foods and those especially which remain in the upper gut and cannot digest but there produce harmful and thick humours. Leek and cabbage and all those which are similarly harsh are to be avoided and that the patient do not lie supine in bed by day and chill and wind and smoke and dust; these things and those like them every day injure the eyes.'

Oribasius, *Synopses* V.33: 'For cloudiness of the eyes. That they should not suffer dimness of the eyes and when they immerse themselves in cold water (they should hold the eyes open in it for a long time), they are able to see things further. Nor does it impede the sight for reading, for the ability is increased by it. To be mistrusted are much and sweet wine and sweet things and foods which remain much in the upper parts of the gut and indigested and generate humid and fat materials, and let them avoid rocket, leek and whatever things are harsh, and let them not lie supine in bed during the day; and cold and wind are injurious and smoke and dust.'[36]

[33] 'Ad caliginem oculorum. Herbae celidoniae sucus vel flos eius expressus et mixtus cum melle attico in vaso aereo, leniter cineri ferventi commixtus decoctusque singulare remedium contra caliginem oculorum. Quidam suco tantum utuntur.'

[34] 'Sucus florentibus exprimitur et in aereo vase cum melle attico leniter cinere ferventi decoquitur singulari remedio contra caligines oculorum.'

[35] 'Item ruta siluestre cum ros suum tundens et sucum eius cum melle dispumatum mittis paris ponderis et inunguis; mirifice prodest.'

[36] 'Ad nebula oculorum. Ut autem non patiuntur caliginem oculi, et quando mergent si [*read* se] in aqua frigida [*'old' Latin version and Greek add*: diu in eadem oculis apertis intendant]; longius uidere possunt in uisum. Non enim inpedit ad legendum visio; additus enim ex hoc uirtus. In suspitionem sit vinus multus et dulces et cibos qui in superiora ventris multum manet et indigestis et humida generant opera et pinguis, eruga, porrus, et quaecumque sunt agra fugiant, et lectum supinum non jaceat indini [*'old' Latin version*: diu]; et frigus et ventus contrarius est; et fumo et puluere.'

4. 'For dimness of the eyes; take green fennel, put in water for thirty nights in a crock which has been pitched on the outside, then fill with rain water, after that throw away the fennel and each day wash the eyes with the water and open them.'

Oribasius, *Synopses*, V.33: 'And as treatment for ailments of the eyes every day do this: put green fennel in water for thirty-one days in an earthen container pitched on the outside with pitch (let the water be rainwater), and after the fennel has been discarded wash the eyes with the water daily, bathe them open [reading *apertum* for *aptum*].'[37]

5. 'Again: from inflammatory vapour and exhalation and from nausea comes dimness of the eyes and the sharpness and eructation cause that. This is to be done for it: For dimness of the eyes take celandine juice a spoonful, another of fennel [juice], a third of southernwood juice, and of virgin honey two spoonfuls, mix together, and then with a feather put on the eyes in the morning and when it is midday and again at evening, after it has become dried and exhausted. Because of the sharpness of the salve, take the milk of a woman who has a child, put in the eyes.'

Physica Plinii 17.1: 'The vapour of choler makes a curse, of which the sharpness brings dimness to the eyes; for which make thus: mix together juice of the herb celandine and of fennel or of southernwood two spoonfuls, of it spread on with a feather in the morning and after noon and at evening, and after digestion; pour over it the milk of a woman who nurses a child, on account of the sharpness of the medicine, that it may cool it.'[38]

6. 'Again, a noble recipe: take balsam and virgin honey, equal amounts of both, mix together and anoint with that.'

Physica Plinii 17.3: 'Again, balsam with virgin honey, mix in equal parts, then put in the eyes.'[39]

7. 'Again for the same: celandine juice and sea-water, anoint the eyes with it and bathe. It is then best that you take the juice of celandine and of mugwort and rue, equal amounts of all, add honey and balsam if you have it, put in a vessel where you may cook it sealed and use; it cures well.'

Physica Plinii 17.8: 'Again, celandine juice (which the eyes support very well) with a collyrium or with sea-water cures in one application; and cooked in water

[37] 'Et cura causa oculorum per singulos dies hoc faciant; aqua triginta et una diebus fenuculum viridem mittes in vaso ceram [*'old' Latin version*: testeo] et deforis picitum de pice; aqua sit pluviales; et projecto fenuculo, de aqua cottidie lauas oculum aptum fouis.'

[38] 'Fumus colerum anathimiasint facit, cuius acritudo caligines oculis prestat; ad quam facies ita: sucus herbe celidonie et fenuculi uel aprotani cocliaria II comisces, exinde ad pinna subfundes mane et post meridies et sero, sed post digestione; lac mulieris que pueru nutrit super fundis propter aceruitate medicamenti, ut refrigere.'

[39] 'Item balsamum cum melle stillaticio equis partibus misces, exinde oculis infundis.'

85

paining eyes are bathed with it. Better, if its juice with the juices of mugwort and rue in equal amounts are cooked in water with honey and balsam; for it does wonderfully.'[40]

8. 'For dimness of the eyes: salt burned and rubbed up and mixed with bumblebees' honey; anoint with that.'
   Physica Plinii 17.11: 'Again, roasted salt ground, mixed with Attic honey, removes dimness of the eyes.'[41]

9. 'Again: juice of fennel and roses and rue and bumblebees' honey and kid's gall mixed together, anoint the eyes with that.'
   No source/analogue found.

10. 'Again: green coriander rubbed up and mixed with woman's milk, lay over the eyes.'
    Physica Plinii 13.9: 'Again: green coriander rubbed up, mixed with woman's milk, anoint and place on swollen eyes.'[42]

11. 'Again: take hare's gall and anoint with it.'
    Physica Plinii 18.3: 'Again: anoint frequently with hare's gall, and it removes the dimness.'[43]

12. 'Again: live winkles burned to ashes and mix the ashes with bumblebees' honey.'
    Pliny, *HN* XXIX.119: 'Also to burn live snails (cockles) and to anoint with their ashes with Cretan honey is very useful for dimness.'[44]

13. 'Again: melt in the sun the fats of all river fishes and mix with honey, anoint with it.'
    Marcellus, *De medicamentis* 138.9: 'The fats of all river fishes melted in the sun and anointed on with honey added to form an ointment is marvellously good for dimness of the eyes.'[45]

---

[40] 'Item celidonie sucum – que oculi plurimum suffragantur – cum collirio siue aqua marina in una unctione sanat; et in aqua decocta dolitantes oculi fobentur. Melius, si succus eius cum artemisie et rute sucis paris portionibus ex melle et balsamo intras aqua coquatur: mire enim facit.'

[41] 'Item sal frixum tritum admixtum melle attico inunctum caliginem tollit.'

[42] 'Item coriandrum uiridem trito admixto lacte mulieris inunguis et super tumentes oculos inpones.'

[43] 'Item de fel leporinum subinde inungue, et caliginem tollit.'

[44] '(Cocleas) vivas quoque cremare et cinere earum cum melle Cretico inunguere caligines utilissimum est.'

[45] 'Adipes omnium fluuialium piscium in sole liquefactae adiunctoque melle inunctioni adhibitae mirifice oculis caligantibus prosunt.'

Pliny, *HN* XXXII.69: 'The fats of all river and marine fishes melted in the sun and mixed with honey confers clearness to the eyes very well.'[46]

14. 'For dimness of the eyes again: betony juice beaten with its roots and wrung out and juice of yarrow and celandine, equal amounts of all, mix together, put in the eyes.'
No source/analogue found.

15. 'Again: fennel roots pounded, mix with pure honey, boil then over a light fire carefully to the thickness of honey, then put in a brass ampulla and when there is need anoint with it; this drives away dimnesses of the eyes even though they are thick.'
Marcellus, *De medicamentis* 136.5: 'Mix with the juice of bruised fennel root the same amount of the best strained honey, preferably Attic, and cook it down over a slow fire to the thickness of honey, and keep it stored up in a brass [copper] box. When there is need, anoint it on with well-water or woman's milk; even if they are thick it disperses obscurities quickly.'[47]

16. 'For dimness of the eyes again: the juice of celandine or its blossoms, strain and mix with bumblebees' honey, put in a brass vessel, then make lukewarm carefully in warm coals or in ashes until it is done; this is a salutary treatment for dimness of the eyes. Some use the juice alone and anoint the eyes with it.'
Herbarium 75.2: 'For dimness of the eyes. Juice of the herb celandine or its flower expressed and mixed with Attic honey in a brass vessel, mixed together and cooked slowly over hot coals is a singular remedy for dimness of the eyes. Some use the juice alone.'[48]

17. 'For dimness of the eyes again: Earth-ivy juice and fennel juice, put equal amounts of both in an ampulla, then dry in the hot sun and anoint the eyes inwardly with it.'
No source/analogue found.

18. 'For dimness of the eyes again: the juice of centaury, that is herdwort, anoint on the eyes; the sight will be sharper for it. If you add honey that is good.'
Physica Plinii 17.10: 'Again: the juice of the lesser centaury with honey added in

---

[46] 'Omnium piscium fluviatilium marinorumque adipes liquefacti sole admixto melle oculorum claritati plurimum conferunt.'

[47] 'Feniculi radicis contusae suco tantundem mellis optimi despumati utinam Attici misceto eaque lento igne ad mellis crassitudinem discoquito repositaque in pyxide etiam aerea habeto. Cum erit opus, cum aqua cisternina aut muliebri lacte inungueto; quamuis crassas caligines cito discuties.'

[48] 'Ad caliginem oculorum. Herbae celidoniae sucus vel flos eius expressus et mixtus cum melle attico in vaso aereo, leniter cineri ferventi commixtus decoctusque singulare remedium contra caliginem oculorum. Quidam suco tantum utuntur.'

equal amounts, mixed and anointed on reduces dimness; and the eyes are bathed with the cooked water itself.'[49]

Herbarium 36.2: 'For decreasing sharpness of the eyes. The juice of the herb the lesser centaury reduces the sharpness of the eyes, they are healed, also with honey added the same is brought about, also with dimness of the eyes so that clearness is restored.'[50]

19. 'Then take a good handful of the same herb, put in a jugful of wine and boil 'ofnete' three days beforehand, and when it is cooked strain off the herb, and sweeten the liquid with honey, drink a bowlful every day after the night's fast.'

Marcellus, *De medicamentis*, 136.10: 'Sharper vision is restored to dim eyes, nor does one fall easily into this complaint who uses such a remedy as a clean handful of centaury in the best wine, but puts it in a new congium or also boils it up and three days macerates in a sealed or closed container, then after three days drinks daily fasting an emina of its wine mixed with hot water with honey added, the centaury remaining in it.'[51]

Physica Plinii 17.10: 'Again: for dimness of the eyes so that clearness may be restored and that this danger may not happen easily: a handful of the herb centaury is cooked in six sesters of wine, macerated for three days; it is taken out, then an emina mixed with honey is given to one fasting daily.'[52]

Borrowings such as we find here would imply, according to my earlier assumption, that they were made directly by the compiler of the *Leechbook* from Latin medical works which he had to hand. But because of Meaney's valuable work on variant versions of Old English remedies, we must be cautious in making inferences of this kind; the most we can infer is that these Latin works were known to the Anglo-Saxons by the end of the ninth century and that probably, but by no means certainly, some of them were in Bald's possession. I will summarize enough of Meaney's evidence to

[49] 'Item centaurie minoris sucus adiecto melle equis portionibus permixtus et inunctus caliginem extenua; et ipsa aqua decocta oculi fobentur.'

[50] 'Ad oculorum aciem deponendam. Herbae centuriae minoris sucus oculis inunctus aciem extenuat, sanantur, adiecto etiam melle idem proficit, caliginantibus quoque oculis ut claritas restituatur.'

[51] 'Caliginantibus oculis uisus acutior restituetur neque facile in hoc uitium incidet, qui usus fuerit remedio tali, ut centaureae manipulum nitidum in uini optimi, sed nouellastri congium mittat aut etiam excoquat ac triduo in uasculo clauso uel operto macerari faciat, deinde post triduum heminam eius uini mixtam cum calida aqua adiecto melle ieiunus manente illic centaurea cottidie bibat.'

[52] 'Item caliginantibus oculis ut claritas restituatur et ne facilem hoc periculum incidant: centaurie herbe manipulum in uino ʃʃ VI coquitur hac triduo maceratur; eximitur, inde cotidie emina mixta melle ieiuno propinnatur.'

show why we must exercise such caution in assigning ownership of Latin medical manuscripts to any single individual.[53]

In 1562 Laurence Nowell transcribed the manuscript subsequently entered in Cotton's library as Otho B. xi which was largely destroyed in the fire at Ashburnham House in 1731. In Nowell's transcript (now London, BL, Add. 43703) the last item is a collection of medical recipes, most of which are also in Bald's *Leechbook*. On 262v we find the following (I have numbered Nowell's entries to correspond to the numbers in the *Leechbook* transcript above):

(1) Wiþ eagena miste. Genim celeþonian seau oþþe blosman gemeng wiþ dorena hunig gedo in æren fæt wlece listum in wearmum gleadum oþþæt hit gesoden sie þis *wið eagena miste.*

(16) Wiþ eagena miste. Eft celeþonian seaw oþþe þara blostmana gewring 7 gemeng wiþ dorena hunig gedo in æren fæt wlece þonne listum in wearmum gledum oððe in æscan oðþæt hit gedon sie. þæt byþ anspilde lyb wiþ eagna dimnesse. Sume þæs seawes anlypies nyttiað 7 þa eagan þi smiriað.

(17) Eft eorþifigis seaw 7 finoles gedo bega efenfeala 7 in ampulan dryge þonne in hatre sunnan 7 þa eagan inanweard mid þy smirige.

(18) Eft wiþ eagena miste eorþgeallan seaw þæt is hyrdewyrt smire in þa eagan sio sien biþ þy scea[r]pre. Gif þu hunig tu dest þæt deah.

(19) Genim þonne þære ilcan wyrte godene gelm gedo in ceac fulne wines 7 geseoð oþþe nete ær iii dagas. Ond þonne hio gesoden sie awring þa wyrt þurh clað of 7 þæs woses geswettes mid hunie gedrince ælce dæge niht nistig bollan fulne.[54]

Meaney has pointed out that the apparent confusion at the end of remedy (1) of Nowell's transcript, where it ends incomplete with the word 'þis' followed by the words 'wið eagena miste' which were first written in and then crossed out and followed immediately by the second version (16) of the same remedy, indicates a problem in his exemplar. She writes:

When we turn to the parallel remedies in Bald's *Leechbook* we find that the remedy at the top of [Nowell's 262v] is the first in [*Leechbook*] 1, ch. ii, on eye ailments, and ends *þis bið god læcedom wiþ eagena dimnesse* . . ., and then follows with many more recipes for the same . . . before reaching the remedy which in Nowell is second on 262v, and continuing with the rest of those on the page. Surely, then, Nowell's *þis* must have been the last word on one sheet, and the following *wiþ eagena miste* the heading at the top of another, but in between there must originally

53 Meaney, 'Variant Versions', *passim.*
54 I have transcribed these directly from the manuscript, London, BL, Add. 43703.

have been one or two sheets which did not survive to be copied into Otho [Nowell's exemplar].[55]

She also pointed out that the two versions of the remedy (1 and 16) vary enough in both the *Leechbook* and in Nowell's transcript that we can be sure that, although both of them may have come ultimately from the *Herbarium* or from Pliny, they were copied from different translations, and that the differences between the *Leechbook* entries and Nowell's show that neither was copied from the other's exemplar.

It follows that if neither collection was copied from the other, then neither need be an original selection or translation of remedies by their compilers; that is, the entries of the *Leechbook* which are also found in Nowell need not have been selected and translated from Latin originals by the compiler of the *Leechbook*, so that we cannot claim that he had copies of the works of Pliny and Marcellus and Oribasius before him as he worked. What we can say is that, if he did not have them, someone before him had access to them, so that Anglo-Saxons had in their libraries the works (or extracts from them) which we find used as sources for these entries in the *Leechbook*. Bald himself may have had them too, but the evidence does not permit us to say so.

This comparison of the *Leechbook* and Nowell versions of this group of remedies also shows that there were recipe collections in English older than either from which both took material and that both did not draw from the same exemplar, as witness the corrupt word *ofnete* in the *Leechbook* and *oppenete* in the same position in Nowell's transcript. This implies that the translation of this recipe had been copied often enough for not one but two corrupt forms to have appeared. Moreover, there still exists another document that leads to the same conclusion that there were Old English medical texts in existence quite some time before the compilation of the *Leechbook*.

I have listed among Old English medical texts (above, p. 31) the Omont fragment, a single leaf containing on the recto only several recipes dealing with ailments of the foot, leg and thigh and with paralysis, and have suggested that it may be a last leaf of a recipe collection. The fragment has been dated to the last half of the ninth century and placed in a centre under Mercian influence. That is, it may be up to half a century older than the exemplar of the *Leechbook* and of a different provenance. Some of its

---

[55] Meaney, 'Variant Versions', pp. 248–9.

recipes are also found in the *Leechbook*, but it is clear that neither text is a source of the other. For example, the Omont fragment has a recipe for a powder to put on wounds: 'Make a good powder for a rotting wound. Take oak bark and the inner bark of sloethorn root. Dry, work to a powder. It is good to sprinkle on the wound.'[56] The similar one in Bald's *Leechbook* reads: 'Again, a good wound salve: oak bark, dry the bark and pound it very fine and dig up the lower part of sloethorn, shave the uppermost bark and pound very fine, sift small through a small sieve, take equal amounts of both; the meal is good to sprinkle on.'[57] Meaney has pointed out that, although these are two forms of a single remedy, they differ in several details. Omont requires the inner bark of sloethorn root, *Leechbook* the uppermost; Omont gives it as a remedy for a rotting wound, *Leechbook* does not specify a particular kind; Omont gives a very brief method of preparation, *Leechbook* is detailed and repetitive. These differences and others in other shared recipes make it clear that the two were compiled from different sources, again implying that there were vernacular collections, now lost, older than either and that there were variant versions of these older collections.

Before we leave this group of *Leechbook* remedies we should consider a few other inferences which can be drawn from them. No sources or analogues have been found for numbers 9, 14 and 17. Remedy 9 requires gall of a kid; Old English remedies requiring medicines from goats are few and most of them can be traced to sources/analogues in the Latin literature. This implies that remedy 9 also may have a Mediterranean origin and that earlier than the time these recipes were borrowed, the goat had not been sufficiently common among the Anglo-Saxons for them to have developed native medicines from it. Remedy 17 contains the Latin word *ampulla* implying translation from a Latin text, so that it also may be of Mediterranean origin. On the other hand, all the ingredients in remedy 14 are plants which grow freely in Britain and Northern Europe, so that it may be of native origin. This somewhat unsatisfactory kind of reasoning can be

---

[56] Schaumann and Cameron, 'A Newly-Found Leaf', lines 289–312: 'Wyrc god dust to rotigendun dolge. Nim acrinde ⁊ slahðornes wyrtruman rinde innewarde. Adryg, wyrc to duste. ðæt bið god in dolg to scædenne.' The fragment has been moved to another library and is now: Louvain-la-Neuve, Université Catholique de Louvain, centre Général de Documentation, Fragmenta H. Omont 3.

[57] *Leechdoms*, ed. Cockayne II, 92–4: 'Eft dolhsealf god: acrind, adrige þa rinde ⁊ swiðe smale gecnuwa ⁊ adelf niþeweardne slahðorn, ascaf þa yfemestan rinde ⁊ swiðe smale gecnuwa, asift smale þurh smæl sife, do begea emfela, þæt mela bið god on to sceadenne.'

applied to any entry in the Anglo-Saxon texts, although it allows us only to guess at origins where sources/analogues have not been found.

The other remedies of the group have analogues in Pliny, Marcellus, Oribasius, *Physica Plinii* and the *Herbarium*. They supply excellent evidence that the *Physica Plinii* was well known to the Anglo-Saxons, it being the most probable source for so many of the entries especially as so many are grouped in the same fashion in the *Leechbook* as in the *Physica Plinii*: apparently these were transferred *en bloc*. The surviving Old English version of the *Herbarium* was not used for remedies borrowed from the *Herbarium*, as all their translations differ. Entries 3 and 4 give further evidence for the popularity of the works of Oribasius in England. We have seen earlier that the *Euporistes* was known, and here we find the *Synopsis*.

From the quotations from these two works in the *Leechbook*, we can learn something about the Latin version from which they were made. The *Euporistes* and *Synopsis* were translated twice into Latin and it used to be believed that one of them, the 'old' one, was made in the sixth century or early seventh and the other, the 'new' one, as late as the tenth. Mørland has shown convincingly, from internal evidence, that both translations are of the same age and that differences in language reflect contemporary usages in Southern and Northern Italian schools and that both translations can be assigned to the late sixth or early seventh century.[58] All quotations from Oribasius in the *Leechbook* can be traced to the 'new' translation, thus offering independent confirmation for Mørland's dating.

It may not always be possible, when a remedy has been traced to Latin sources, to be sure from which source it was taken. Writers of Latin medical works borrowed freely from one another and the English compiler may have had the opportunity to take his remedy from more than one of these works. The *Herbarium* is almost certainly the direct source of remedy 1 and of the almost identical remedy 16, but both might have come from Pliny instead, depending on how many intermediate copyings may have been made between the first borrowing and the final entry in the *Leechbook*, each copying giving opportunity for changes in wording which would conceal the details of an originally close translation. Similarly, remedy 18 may have come equally well from *Physica Plinii* or the *Herbarium*, and since both source texts were available to the Anglo-Saxons

[58] H. Mørland, 'Die lateinischen Oribasiusübersetzungen', *Symbolae Osloenses*, Supplementum 5 (Oslo, 1932).

there is no reason to prefer one over the other. On the other hand, remedies 13 and 19 were almost certainly taken from the work of Marcellus, because they resemble his text much more closely than any of the alternative ones.

It is in bk II that Bald's *Leechbook* demonstrates its superiority over the general run of medical texts of its time and later. Two very interesting quotations from the *Epitome altera* of Vindicianus introduce groups of chapters on diseases of the liver and of the spleen. The one on the liver allows a rare insight into the physiological ideas of the Middle Ages:

It (the liver) is extended on the right side as far as the flank, it has five lobes, is connected with the loins, is the building material and dwelling-place of the blood and its nourishment; when there is digestion and liquefaction of foods they come to the liver, then they change their form and turn into blood, and it removes the impurities which are there and collects the clean blood and sends it out chiefly through four blood vessels to the heart and also through all the body as far as the extremities of the limbs.[59]

This is a close translation of parts of the corresponding chapter of the *Epitome*:

Our liver is situated on the right side extended as far as the large gut, that is parts of the flank. It has five lobes, bordering upon the kidneys and the right flank and with the liver also the green bladder, that is bile. *The liver is the peculiar material and seat of the blood and its increase. For there the thin consistency of foods is changed with a change of colour into blood.* All the matter of foods broken up through the windpipe [?oesophagus] is sent first of all from the stomach, and is distributed through all the body by very slender routes. Therefore the liver sends it out into the blood very green and in very good condition. *Then what are most foul and in its opinion to be rejected are discharged* into the belly, the intestines are filled, *the liver accepts the most foul parts from food and cooking them with its heat liquefies them at length. From this it makes blood, which first it collects with many pipes. then taken up it is led to four major blood vessels* which are to the liver like a reservoir. For it has two receptacles in itself,

59 *Leechdoms*, ed. Cockayne II, 198: 'Sio (þa lifer) biþ on þa swiþran sidan aþened oþ þone neweseoþan sio hæfð fif læppan helt þa lendenbrædan sio is blodes timber 7 blodes hus 7 foster þonne þara metta meltung biþ 7 þynnes þa becumaþ on þa lifer þonne wendaþ hie hiora hiw 7 cerrað on blod 7 þa unsefernessa þe þær beoþ hio awyrpþ ut 7 þæt clæne blod gesomnaþ 7 þurh feower ædra swiþost onsent to þære heortan 7 eac geond ealne þone lichoman oþ þa ytmestan limo.'

one breath, the other vital principle, that is blood, through which, as I said, nine arteries for breath enter the body and four blood vessels go out. Therefrom, very large and by its own growth become greater and greater, *it goes to the extremeties of the members* and produces the pulse.[60]

The borrowing is as interesting for what it adds to its source as for what it leaves out. The *Leechbook* does not mention the gall bladder, and the *Epitome* does not mention the heart; in many ways the Old English account is clearer and closer to the actual physiological situation. The idea that the liver manufactures blood is the most obvious error of both accounts.

The compiler's use of Vindicianus's account of the spleen follows much the same procedure; the *Leechbook* reads

How the spleen is oblong and connected to the gut: It has a thin membrane, which has fat and thick veins, and the membrane is a protector and encloses the gut and the bowels and warms them, and is extended on the left flank and is confined by sinewy branches, and on the one side is broad, reaching the side, on the other in contact with the innards. About laughter which comes from the spleen: some say that the spleen is subject to the sinews and that the spleen in some parts is dead or absent in people and that for that reason they can laugh.[61]

Vindicianus wrote:

---

[60] *Theodori Prisciani Euporiston. etc*, ed. Rose, pp. 474–5: '*Epar nostrum ponitur in dextro latere extensum usque ad langaones hoc est ilium eius partes. Pinnas habet quinque, continens renes et ilia dextra* et iocinere et uissica uiride hoc est fel. *Est autem iecor propria materia sanguinis domus et incrementum eius. Nam ibi tenuitas ciborum mutato colore transfiguratur in sanguine.* Omnis autem materia ciborum detunsa per gurgulionem excipitur primo ab stomacho. Que tenuissima itinera per totum corpus dispensatur. Ergo uiridissima et integerrima in sanguinem dimittit iecor. *Tunc que sordidissima et iudicis suo reprobata sunt*, exonerantur in uentrem, intestines repletantur, *accipit iecor sordidissima ex cibo et illa calore suo tam diu decoquendo liquescit. Inde sanguinem fit, quem primum multis colligit fistolis, deinde acceptum maioribus uenulis quatuor perducitur* que ad iecor quasi ad castellum. Duo enim receptacula intra se habet, unum spiritus, alterum anima, hoc est sanguis, per cuius, ut dixi, corpore ut arterias spiritales nouem intrant et quattuor exeunt uene sanguinales. Inde immensus et suo sibi incremento maior atque maior factus, *extremis usque ad finem membrorum emigat* redditque pulsum.'

[61] *Leechdoms*, ed. Cockayne II, 242: 'Hu se milte bið emlang 7 gædertenge þære wambe hæfð þynne filmene sio hæfð fætte 7 þicce ædra 7 sio filmen biþ þeccende 7 weronde þa wambe 7 þa innefaran 7 þa wyrmð 7 is aþened on þone winestran neweseoþan 7 is mid sinehtum limum gehæfd 7 is on oðre healfe brad gehrineð þære sidan on oðre is ðam innoðe getang. Be hleahtre þe of milte cymð sume secgaþ þæt se milte ðam sinum þeowige 7 þætte se milte on sumum dælum þam monnum adeadige oþþe of sie 7 þæt hi for þon hylhhan mægen.'

The spleen is situated on the left side of the midriff, oblong in shape. It is attached to the belly. It has on its outside a thin membrane and a covering having very stout veins, which either envelopes or warms the belly, and which the Greeks call epiplos [ἐπίπλοος]. In Latin it is called the omentum or mappa. *It is spread out as far as the left flank and placed [over] the gut, which is held by sinewy membranes. On one side it is flat and touches the side, on the other it adheres to the viscera,* and on that account as it usually happens, a particular impediment to those running, so that when a swelling has adhered it to anything, it causes very sharp pains of the whole part of the body covering the nearest parts of the left side, nor does it easily abate from that incapacity, since it is held together by material and sinewy bonds. *It is taught by some that the spleen is served by the kidneys and they are augelotus [ἀγελώτος], (except for those in whom part of the spleen may be dead or absent), they are not able to laugh.*[62]

The Old English account of the spleen deals only with its position in the abdomen and its relation to other organs, leaving out all of the original's comments on various names, symptoms, etc. The final sentence needs further comment; the spleen was once supposed to be the seat of melancholy and so inimical to laughter unless a part of it was non-functional or lacking, when laughter was possible. This property of the spleen was described by Vindicianus as 'augelotus', ignored by the translator who most likely did not understand it, the Greek ἀγελώτος ('unable to laugh') being an unusual word.

One gets the impression that turning Latin medical terms into Old English must have been a problem. This is most noticeable in Bald's *Leechbook*, where translation was from highly technical articles, and so various strategies were employed. The translator often used a Latin loanword even when an Old English equivalent was available: *cancer adl, þæt is bite* for 'cancer'; *paralysin, þæt is on englisc lyft adl* for 'paralysis'.[63] This was not a common practice, *lyft adl* being the usual translation for 'paralysis'.

[62] *Theodori Prisciani Euporiston, etc.*, ed. Rose, pp. 475–6: '*Splen autem ponitur in sinistra parte precordiorum, natura oblongus. Coniunctus est uentri. Continet ex se membranam tenuem et uelamen habens pinguissimas uenas, que uentrem uel intestinas cooperit uel calefacit,* quod Graeci epiplos uocant. Latine omentum uel mappa dicitur. *Extensum est usque ad ilium sinistrum et interanea positus, quod neruosis continetur membranis. Ab una parte planus est latus contingit, ab altera uisceribus adherit,* ideoque ut fieri solet, peculiare inpedimentum currentibus, ut cum tumor ille aliquis inhesit, aceruissimos dolores totius partis corporis sinistriores extensus proximietates efficit, nec facile inbecillitate remittit. Quoniam ipse fungi de materiae et neruosis continetur uinculis. *Traditur a quibusdam spleni renibus deseruire et esse augelotus, quibus autem mortua pars spleni sit aut exemta, ridere posse negantur.*'

[63] *Leechdoms*, ed. Cockayne II, 10 and 108 (*cancer adl*); 12 (*paralysin*).

More commonly existing English terms were used: *geoxa* for *singultus*; *geswel þæt is aþundenes* for *flegmon id est tumor iecoris*; *healfdes heafdes ece* for *emigranium*; *hwosta* for *tussis*; *maga* for *stomachus*; *milte* for *splen*; *oman* for *erysipelas*; *wæta* for *humor*; *wamb* for *uenter*; *wlætta* for *nausea*; *wund þære lifre* for *elcosis id est uulneratio iecoris*.[64] Where the Latin text had explained a Greek term by a Latin gloss (*flegmon*, *elcosis*), the English writer translated the Latin gloss. Sometimes he used an English term having the same primary meaning as the Latin term, although both were used in derived senses: the primary meaning of both *singultus* and *geoxa* is 'sob'; 'hiccough' is secondary in both languages. *Humor* and *wæta* both mean 'dampness', 'moisture'; 'physiological humour' is a derived meaning. *Oman*, used to translate *erysipelas*, is a derivative of *om* ('rust'), probably because of the deep red colour of the skin in erysipelatous infections. Some terms, such as *maga*, *milte* and *wamb*, were native anatomical words in general use long before they were given any special medical connotations.

The compiler of Bald's *Leechbook* used some Old English terms with meanings not found elsewhere: *neweseoþa* for *ilium* and *wang* (*weng*, *wæng*) for *frons*.[65] *Neweseoþa* usually means 'pit of the belly' ('stomach') rather than, as in the *Leechbook*, 'flank'. Elsewhere in Old English *wang* means 'cheek';[66] only in the *Leechbook* does it stand for 'forehead'. Latin and Modern English equivalents have not been found for all Old English medical terms and there are others for which suggested meanings are doubtful. *Fic* usually means fig-like outgrowths, such as haemorrhoids, styes on the eye or the papules on the inner side of the eyelid in trachomatous conditions. But what does it mean in the following: 'Wiþ seondum omum . . . þæt is fic' ('For oozing erysipelas . . . that is, *fic*')?[67] Fig-like outgrowths do not seem a likely accompaniment of a weeping ulcer. Another difficult term is *þeor* or *þeoradl*, frequently used for what seems most often to be some rashy or eruptive skin condition, as well as ailments of the respiratory structures. *Hreofl* ('scabbiness') and *micel lic* ('big body') cannot be accurately interpreted; *hreofl* is usually translated 'leprosy', yet it is not at all clear that the leprosy of ancient and medieval medicine was confined to Hansen's disease, but was also used to designate

---

[64] *Ibid.*, pp. 60 (*geoxa*), 198 (*geswel*), 20 (*healfdes heafdes ece*), 56 (*hwosta*), 174 (*maga*), 242 (*milte*), 98 (*oman*), 60 (*wæta*), 220 (*wamb*), 62 (*wlætta*), and 198 (*wund þære lifre*).

[65] *Ibid.*, pp. 198, 258 (*neweseoða*) and 20 (*weng*).

[66] See, for example, *Leechbook III* (*ibid.* II, 338).

[67] *Ibid.*, II, 102.

cutaneous conditions with an appearance similar to that of true leprosy. *Micel lic*, although usually translated by 'elephantiasis', probably designated other conditions manifesting an enlargement of bodily tissues (including the skin) as well, such as von Recklinghausen's disease or even acromegaly. *Micel lic* is mentioned in several remedies in the *Leechbooks* but it is not likely that filiarial infections (the usual cause of true elephantiasis) leading to enlargement of lymphatic tissues should have been found in England. Other terms which describe ailments which cannot be certainly identified now are *feondes costung* ('demon's temptation'), *ælfadl* ('elfsickness'), *deofolseocnes* ('demon sickness') and *wæterælfadl* ('waterelfsickness', 'chicken pox'), simply because we do not know to what extent these terms were used literally or were left-overs from a time when devils and elves were supposed to cause illnesses, just as one today does not associate astrology with the disease called *influenza* ('influence (of the stars)') nor do speakers of German think of witches when they call lumbago *Hexenschuss* (witch-shot'). It must also be borne in mind that it is exceedingly difficult and often misleading to attempt diagnoses or identifications of diseases when the information is as scanty as it frequently is in ancient and medieval medical records.

Translations were sometimes ambiguous or misleading and sometimes wrong. The compiler of Bald's *Leechbook* regularly gave *laures croppan* ('laurel bunches') for *bacas lauri* (*cropp* can mean 'sprout', 'berry', 'flower', etc.); he gave *pysena seaw* ('juice of peas') and *geseawe pysan* ('juicy peas') for *ptisane succos* ('barley broths' or 'barley water'), but this may have resulted from errors in his exemplars; he translated *cardiaca passio* ('dyspepsia', 'heartburn') by *heortcoþu* ('heart ailment'); the Latin term is a literal translation of the Greek καρδιακὴ διάθεσις, which refers to the cardiac region of the stomach, the 'mouth of the stomach'.[68] That either the Latin or English translators knew this we have no way of knowing; today *heartburn* evokes not a picture of heart disease but rather that of a burning sensation in the oesophagus. It is sometimes difficult to see how the translator could have made some of his errors unless he was working from defective exemplars; for example: 'All broth is to be abstained from because

---

[68] *Leechdoms*, ed. Cockayne II, 20 and elsewhere (*laures croppan*), 246 and 254 (*pysena seaw* and *geseawe pysan*), 176 (*heortcoþu*). For further comment on 'heortcoþu', see W. Bonser, 'Anglo-Saxon Medical Nomenclature', *English and German Studies* 4 (1951–2), 13–19.

it is inflating and causes harmful humours.'[69] This statement comes in the midst of a long and otherwise well-translated passage from the *Practica Alexandri*, where the corresponding passage reads: 'Therefore there is to be given barley broth which can evacuate and relax constipated places and mitigate burning inflammation.'[70]

An interesting mistake in translation occurs in the first chapter of bk II of the *Leechbook*.[71] In a list of foods suitable for an ailing stomach, Alexander gave ἰσικοί ('minced meat', 'hash'), which in *Practica Alexandri* was transliterated as 'ysicia'.[72] The word obviously puzzled the Anglo-Saxon translator, who took it to be a form of the Latin *esox* which then designated the salmon, for he translated it by *leax* ('salmon'). Indeed, he seems to have recognized (incorrectly) only the word *ysicia* in a long list of foods which digest slowly: 'de piscibus bulbia et pectines et astaci et ysicia de pectine et cyritia', which, by the way, is a quite inaccurate Latin rendering of Alexander's Greek original, where the first two items, βοῦλβα and στέρνιον, were not fishes but 'sowbellies' and 'spare-ribs'. As far as it concerned diet, it probably did not make much difference to a patient which he was given to eat.

Interesting is the disease *bite* which was equated with the Latin *cancer*. Pauline Thompson has shown that *bite* and *cancer* were so infrequently mentioned in Anglo-Saxon literature that we must suppose true cancer was not a common ailment in England. That either *bite* or *cancer* always meant the same disease as is meant by the modern term *cancer* is very doubtful, although there is no doubt that cancer as we know it was included in the two terms, which also covered any ulcer hard to heal. Thompson suggests reasons why cancer might not be common in Anglo-Saxon England, among which would be a relatively short life expectancy, cancer being primarily a disease of older people.[73]

On the whole, given their wholly inadequate lexical aids, translators of medical works into Old English did a commendable job, one just as good as their Latin predecessors did with their Greek originals. The high level of

---

[69] *Leechdoms*, ed. Cockayne II, 210: 'Ælc broþ is to forganne for þon þe hit biþ þindende 7 swigene.'

[70] *Practica Alexandri* 2.61: 'Dandus est ergo sucus ptisane qui proiicere et relaxare constipata loca possit et ardentem temperare flegmonem.'

[71] *Leechdoms*, ed. Cockayne II, 176. [72] *Practica Alexandri* 2.14.

[73] P. Thompson, 'The Disease that we Call Cancer', *Health, Disease and Healing in Medieval Culture*, ed. S. Campbell, B. Hall and D. Klausner (New York, 1992), pp. 1–11.

organization of Bald's *Leechbook* implies an equally high level of organization of materials before they were entered in the book. There must have been some kind of 'card-indexing' system. Audrey Meaney, commenting on the composition of the Otho collection of recipes, now almost all lost, has made a point which can equally well apply to Bald's collection and which would explain his good organization: 'It is very tempting to postulate that, as remedies came to the compiler's hand, they were copied on to scraps of varying sizes and even varying shapes. Surely every scriptorium must have used offcuts from the edges of expensive and elaborately prepared (but irregularly shaped) skins for their rough work.'[74] There seems to be very little new under the sun. Whatever the method used, there is little duplication in the book and little evidence of disruption of plan.

[74] Meaney, 'Variant Versions', p. 253.

11

Materia medica

The Lord hath created medicines out of the
earth; and he that is wise will not abhor them.[1]

To appreciate the pharmaceutical resources and *materia medica* of the
Anglo-Saxons, answers to certain questions must be sought: (1) What
substances were prescribed in remedies? (2) Were these substances obtainable in England at that time? (3) What was the therapeutic value of these
substances and could they be expected to have beneficial effects on the
ailments for which they were prescribed? We shall deal with the first two of
these questions in this chapter and discuss the third one in the next two
chapters on rational and magical treatments.

The first thing that strikes one looking at a list of prescribed drugs is
their extraordinarily large number. They are of plant, animal and mineral
origins, but those of plant origin are by far the largest group. In Bald's
Leechbook, bk I, there are over 300, of which about 80 per cent are of plant
origin, and in *Leechbook III* there are more than 250, about 70 per cent of
plant origin. Medicines of animal origin include the flesh and fats of
various mammals, birds, fishes and invertebrates, and bodily products
including butter, milk, cheese, eggs, gall, wool, hair, bone, spittle,
blood, urine and faeces, the last four forming what the Germans have called
a *Dreckapotheke* ('filth pharmacy'). The flesh of animals was used mostly in
special diets; butter, milk, cheese, eggs and gall were common ingredients
in medicines; wool was used as a base for applications; hair and bone were
rarely used, and of *Dreckapotheke* urine and blood were used much more
frequently than faecal matter, spittle being rarely called for. Of mineral

[1] Ecclesiaticus XXXVIII.4.

substances those most often prescribed were iron and copper (usually in the form of salts formed in the metal vessels in which medicines were placed), mercury, sulphur, atramentum (which may be a sulphide of copper or iron), tin, salt, nitre, ammoniac and various 'stones'. But although plants accounted for only 70–80 per cent of drugs, they made up well over 90 per cent of the ingredients in recipes, so that for most purposes Anglo-Saxon medicine was a herbal medicine.

The number of ingredients in the medical texts gives a misleading picture of their use, because most of them appear in only one or two recipes: of 256 in *Leechbook III*, 129 appear once each and 46 more twice each; only 11 are prescribed in 10 or more recipes each. In *Leechbook III*, the four most frequently prescribed substances were water (17 times), milk (21), ale (27) and butter (28). In bk I of Bald's *Leechbook* and in *Leechbook III*, the following plants or plant products appear a total of twelve or more times: ivy (12), coriander (12), smallage (13), pennyroyal (15), hindheal (16), centaury (18), radish (20), barley (20), oak (20), carline thistle (20), attorlothe (corydalis/fumitory) (21), cockle (21), celandine (22), yarrow (27), horehound (30), onions and garlic (31), fennel (31), rue (33), lupin (34), plantain (35), elecampane (36), pepper (37), oil (38), wormwood (40), vinegar (45), bishopswort (46), betony (61), wine (66), ale (83), honey (92). In the same collections the most frequently used animal products were: urines of goat, cattle, hound, child (8 in all), dungs of dove, goat, sheep, horse, cattle, swine, human (20 in all), galls of crab, salmon, cattle, goat, swine, bear, hare (30 in all), eggs (28 in all), milks of goat, sheep, cow, human (42 in all), fats of sheep, cattle, goat, swine, horse, bear, fish, hen, goose, deer (49 in all), butter (94). Pigeon, starling and swallow supplied a few medicines, as did dungbeetles, mealworms, ants, snails and earthworms. Although about fifty animal products are mentioned, most of them occurred in only one, two or three recipes each.

Many substances could not have been obtained from native sources and, if used, must have been imported. An example is pepper, prescribed in 33 recipes in bk I of Bald's *Leechbook* and four times in *Leechbook III*. One is bound to ask: could an Anglo-Saxon physician be expected to have on hand even a part of this large pharmacopoeia, or was the compilation of the recipes containing so many ingredients merely an example of the 'mindless copying' of which scribes are so often accused? To get an answer we must explore various pathways of information and conjecture.

Certainly, no medieval physician could be expected to have access to hundreds of ingredients. Charles Singer was most emphatic about this:

It would be an error to regard all the elaborate prescriptions in these writings as indicating the actual lines of treatment. For practical reasons many of the recipes could not have been prepared. Any leech who claimed that he had so prepared them would have been guilty of fraud. In fact dark age medical manuscripts are partly mere literary material and in places hardly more than scribal exercises. They are always unintelligently copied and the prescriptions are often mere elaborate displays of learning. Many of the remedies that they set forth were certainly unintelligible to the leeches of the time; others involved preparations altogether beyond their meagre technical skills.[2]

But an examination of remedies shows that many are alternatives for a single ailment, so that a physician looking for a treatment would have had a choice and should usually have been able to find one requiring only ingredients that he could obtain. Thus the size of the pharmacopoeia may have been an advantage and the copying of a multitude of remedies, rather than being mindless, may have been an intelligent measure designed to enable physicians working under different conditions to find remedies which they could use. A similar situation prevailed in Mediterranean regions; the Περὶ ἁπλῶν φαρμάκων ('simple medicines') of Dioscorides and the Περὶ εὐπορίστων ('common medicines') of Galen and Oribasius were intended for physicians working in rural districts, where they would be unable to procure all the ingredients given in their more elaborate compilations and easily available only in urban districts.[3] It appears that Anglo-Saxon compilers combined both kinds of manual into a single work.

Although a complete answer to the first question above has not yet been given, we must break off from it to consider the availability of ingredients. What could one expect to find in Anglo-Saxon England; were exotic substances found there? It has been claimed that many of these simply were not available. But consider that pepper was more frequently called for in recipes in bk I of Bald's *Leechbook* than many native substances, being required for 33 of them. This implies that it must have been possible to get pepper without too much difficulty and there is independent evidence that it was fairly common. Sometime before 695, Aldhelm of Malmesbury composed an *enigma* for which pepper is the solution:

---

[2] Grattan and Singer, *Anglo-Saxon Magic*, p. 24.

[3] *Dioscuridis de Materia Medica*, ed. Wellmann III, 149–326; *Galeni Opera Omnia*, ed. Kühn XIV; *Œuvres d'Oribase*, ed. Molinier VI.

I am black on the outside, covered with a wrinkled bark, but yet inside I have a shining pith. I season dainties, feasts of kings and extravagant dishes, also sauces and kitchen stews. But you will find me of no value unless my inwards are crushed for their shining pith.[4]

It would have been purposeless for Aldhelm to pose riddles on subjects which were not known to his contemporaries, so that we must conclude that pepper as a condiment was not confined to the dishes of a king's table, but also appeared in the refectory of a monastery. If the flavouring of sauces and stews with pepper was common enough to serve as a clue to its identification in a riddle before the end of the seventh century, it should not surprise us to find it prescribed in many medical recipes in the ninth. That it was known in monasteries in the eighth century we learn from Cuthbert's account of the last days of Bede, where he tells how Bede bequeathed pepper to his fellows at Jarrow at the time of his death in 735.[5]

From the *Leechbooks* themselves we learn of direct acquaintance with another exotic material, silk from China, beyond the India whence pepper came. Twice in the *Leechbooks* silk is specified for sutures following a surgical operation, in one of them (repair of a harelip) because it would 'rot'.[6] The third reference is more revealing as to the source of the silk, where a person suffering from jaundice is said to be 'as yellow as good silk'.[7] This must be a reference to Chinese silk, because Coan silk is of a pale creamy white colour, not at all the yellowish colour of Chinese silk or a jaundiced body.

If pepper and silk from India and China were used by physicians, we should not be surprised to find other substances from equally far away also available to them. Nor should we give too much weight to the complaint of Bishop Cyneheard of Winchester in the mid-eighth century that the medical texts available in his monastery were of little use because of the numbers of foreign drugs prescribed in them which could not be got at Winchester. Bald's *Leechbook*, which appears to have been compiled at

---

[4] Trans. Lapidge and Rosier, *Aldhelm: the Poetic Works*, p. 78; *Collectiones*, ed. Glorie I, 425: 'Sum niger exterius ruguso cortice tectus,/ Sed tamen interius candentem gesto medullam./ Dilicias, epulas regum luxusque ciborum,/ Ius simul et pulpas battutas condo culinae:/ Sed me subnixum nulla virtute videbus,/ Viscera ni fuerint nitidis quassata medullis.'

[5] *Venerabilis Baedae Opera Historica*, ed. C. Plummer, 2 vols. (Oxford, 1896), I, clx–clxiv; see also lxxvi.

[6] *Leechdoms*, ed. Cockayne II, 56 (repair of harelip) and 358 (suture of abdomen).

[7] *Ibid.*, p. 106.

Winchester in the late ninth century, prescribes many exotic drugs. Being a work highly derivative of Greek, Roman, North African and Byzantine medicine, its compiler must have been faced with Cyneheard's problem. If we examine the book with this problem in mind we find that the compiler used the following strategies: (a) when he transferred a group of recipes to his work he sometimes omitted certain ones of the group; (b) he sometimes omitted certain ingredients from a recipe which he transferred; (c) some recipes he transferred unchanged. Remedies omitted from a group usually contained mostly rarely used exotic ingredients; ingredients omitted from transferred recipes were usually exotic; ingredients in recipes transmitted entire were presumably available in England. It appears further that if an exotic ingredient could be transported without loss of efficacy then it was entered in the Old English compilation. Things used in the dried or preserved state and which did not deteriorate in their natural state were entered. Fruits and herbs useful only in the fresh state or which deteriorated quickly were not entered. From this practice of the compiler of Bald's *Leechbook* we can infer a trade in non-perishable drugs and make an estimate of which drugs the compiler expected to be available in England. Thus we have a clue to the importation of drugs and medical necessities from as far away as India, Indonesia, China, the Moluccas, the Near East and Africa in the time of Alfred the Great.[8]

Bk I of Bald's *Leechbook* is the least derivative part of his compilation and so may be presumed to show the usages most common to English medicine, yet a partial list of imported substances includes aloes, balsam, cassia and cinnamon, galbanum, ginger, incense, mastic, quicksilver (mercury), myrtle and wild olive, pepper and silk. Aloes, balsam, incense, mastic, myrtle and wild olive were from Africa, Arabia and the Near East; mercury came from Spain, the others from the Far East, China, Indonesia, Sri Lanka, the Moluccas. An incident in a saint's life reveals something about the trade in these substances. Some time in the first third of the eighth century Willibald, later to be venerated as a saint, returning from the Holy Land, smuggled balsam through customs control at the port of Tyre.[9] The escapade tells us that at that time the

[8] M. L. Cameron, 'Bald's *Leechbook* and Cultural Interaction in Anglo-Saxon England', *ASE* 19 (1990), 5–12. See also J. M. Riddle, 'The Introduction and Use of Eastern Drugs in the Early Middle Ages', *Archiv für die Geschichte der Medizin* 49 (1965), 185–98.

[9] C. H. Talbot, *The Anglo-Saxon Missionaries in Germany* (London, 1954), p. 170.

trade in drugs and spices was large enough to justify governmental controls by the exporting country; that is, it was a trade large enough to be profitably taxed.

The intermediaries in this trade seem to have been the Arabs, and the main trade route seems to have been the old Spice Route from the Far East to Arabia and the Horn of Africa, thence to Levantine ports such as Tyre and from there to Italian ports, or (for some things) by way of Spain. Some imports such as silk may have come by the land route through Persia and what is now Turkey. It was at this time that the Italian city states gained prominence as European trading centres, Venice being the most important. It is not difficult to imagine comparatively easy passage of goods from there to England. Thus there is no intrinsic improbability in supposing a continuing supply of foreign drugs in Anglo-Saxon England.

The names by which these substances were known in England also give information about their origins and their traders. For some an Arabic name was used, transferred through Greek and Latin; thus the Arabic *alloeh* entered Greek as ἀλόη, to become Latin *aloe* and Old English *alwe*. It is a very old drug in European use and the English got it and its uses through the Greeks and Romans. Although it appears in several English recipes, they are borrowed ones; it did not become a common drug. For other drugs, the Greek (Latin) name was translated: μαστίχη ('mastic') became *hwitcwudu* ('white chewing stuff', 'chewing gum') in English. The centre of production of mastic was the island of Scio in the Greek archipelago (where it is still chewed to sweeten the breath) and it probably did not pass through Arab hands on its way to England. It must have been relatively inexpensive, as it appears to have been sufficiently common in England to have received an English name. Were the Anglo-Saxons also gum chewers?

Two recipes in *Lacnunga* are of special interest. Both are made up from mostly native ingredients and show other traces of native origin. But both also contain foreign ingredients; in one recipe these are aloes, laurel berries, pepper and zedoary (rendered in English as *sidewar*), in the other they are ginger, cinnamon, laurel berries, pyrethrum, zedoary and galingale (rendered in English as *gallenger*).[10] *Lacnunga* is a relatively late compilation, probably a century later than the *Leechbooks*: zedoary and galingale are members of the ginger family from the Far East but were unknown to the Greeks and Romans and were introduced into the West only in

[10] Grattan and Singer, *Anglo-Saxon Magic*, pp. 110 and 114.

medieval times by the Arabs. Yet here they are with other foreign drugs among typically native English ones and compounded according to typically English methods. This implies that before the end of the tenth century newly imported Arab trade goods were so well known in England as to be used in the compounding of native remedies.

Another argument against the ability of the Anglo-Saxon physician to prepare many medicines is the claim that many of the fresh herbs required could not have been grown in England. When this argument was first advanced, no serious work had yet been done on the palaeoclimatology of Britain and scholars were not aware that the climate of England from about 500 to 1200 was warmer and drier than the so-called Little Ice Age which followed and from which we have emerged only in the present century.[11] That the climate then was relatively warm is shown by the number of vineyards listed in the Domesday survey; that we are entering, or have entered, a similar period is shown by the fact that grapes are again being grown for wine in Southern England. That the cultivation of herbs was pursued at that time is clear from Charlemagne's *capitularia* concerning things to be provided on the imperial estates,[12] from the *Hortulus* of Walafrid Strabo[13] and the plan of the physic garden at St Gallen.[14] It is entirely possible that any plant required in the fresh state in an Old English recipe could have been grown outdoors in Southern England, especially as most of them were annuals which would not survive over winter in any case and, if particularly tender, could be expected to mature and provide seed for the next year if grown in sheltered gardens. It is unlikely, then, that any ingredient called for in an Old English medical recipe could not be found in England at one place or another, and on that ground at least preparation of recipes was not beyond the ability of the physician.

The question 'What substances were prescribed in recipes?' can be answered only if we can identify them in modern terms. Substances of

---

[11] H. H. Lamb, 'The Early Medieval Warm Epoch and its Sequel', *Palaeogeography, Palaeoclimatology, Palaeoecology* 1 (1965), 13–37.

[12] *MGH, Leges* I, 180 and 186–7. J. Asch, '"And let the gardener have on his house the Beard-of-Jove"', *Garden Journal* 18 (1968), 134–47, gives the facsimile and translation of the *Capitulare de villis*, with identification of all the plants mentioned in it, and a sketch of the plan of the Benedictine Monastery at St Gallen, showing a plan of the physic garden. See also below, n. 13.

[13] *Hortulus of Walahfrid Strabo*, ed. and trans. R. Payne, with commentary by W. Blunt (Pittsburgh, PA, 1966).

[14] Grattan and Singer, *Anglo-Saxon Magic*, p. 14 (fig. 8).

animal origin present almost no difficulty; only very occasionally is there doubt as to their identity. Substances of mineral origin are also usually identifiable; only in a few instances has there been doubt. For example, Cockayne identified the Old English name *attrum* as *olusatrum*, the plant alexanders (*Smyrnium olusatrum*).[15] This identification is almost certainly wrong, alexanders being little used in medicine and then only as a stomachic and diuretic, whereas the most frequent use for *attrum* in Anglo-Saxon medicine was to treat eye ailments. This indicates that it is to be identified with *atramentum*, shoemaker's blacking, which was used mostly in medicines for the eyes.

Identification of plants can be much more difficult; some editors and commentators have bravely attempted identifications for almost every plant mentioned, others have been more cautious, so that we have on the one hand Cockayne, who made serious, if often erroneous, attempts to give modern equivalents to the Old English plant names, and on the other hand Singer, who listed only twenty-seven Old English plant names whose identification with Linnaean species he thought was 'fairly safe'.[16] Most of us would be less inclusive than Cockayne and less exclusive than Singer, yet in spite of all attempts, the interpretation of many Old English plant names is doubtful or unknown. The Old English botanical lexicon has been assembled and analysed by Peter Bierbaumer in three comprehensive volumes.[17]

One of the most difficult problems in these identifications results from the modern system of naming organisms, codified by Linnaeus in the mid-eighteenth century, according to which each living thing is given a name consisting of two words, the first (a noun) assigns it to a genus of related types and the second (an adjective in agreement with the noun) assigning it to a species within that genus. This system of nomenclature has led to taxonomical arrangements for plants based on principles which purport to show their evolutionary relatedness by employing in large measure a consideration of their reproductive structures and strategies as well as of their morphology. Pre-Linnaean identifications were usually

---

[15] *Leechdoms*, ed. Cockayne III, 312.

[16] Grattan and Singer, *Anglo-Saxon Magic*, pp. 87–8.

[17] P. Bierbaumer, *Der botanische Wortschatz des Altenglischen: I. Das Læceboc; II. Lacnunga, Herbarium Apuleii, Peri Didaxeon; III. Der botanische Wortschatz in altenglischen Glossen*, 3 vols., Grazer Beiträge zur Englischen Philologie 3 (Frankfurt-am-Main, 1975–9).

based on gross morphological appearances only and so implied no evolutionary relations. For example, *nettle* and *dead-nettle* share the name *nettle* because of the similarities in the shape and size of leaves and in habit of growth, no attention being paid to striking differences in structure of flowers and reproductive parts, which show that the nearest English relative of the true nettle is pellitory-of-the-wall (*Parietaria diffusa*) of the family Urticaceae, whereas the nearest relatives of dead-nettle are the mints and other members of the family Labiatae. That is, medieval herbalists, looking at habits of growth and appearances of stems and leaves and perhaps medicinal properties, took dead-nettle to be a kind of nettle without stinging hairs, hence *dead*. This does not imply that the medieval herbalist ever mistook the one for the other; his criteria of identification were different from ours but worked equally well in separating the two types of plants. [18] The example just given shows an extreme case of lumping unlikes together (according to our standards), and it is not difficult now to determine that the plant then called 'red nettle' (*reade netele*) is the one to which we give the Linnaean name *Lamium purpureum*, but because we have been given no details of the relatively small differences separating species of the genus *Urtica*, we cannot decide to which of the native species – *Urtica urens* or *U. dioica* – the word *nettle* (*netele*) refers, or even if it may include the foreign species *U. pillulifera*, introduced into England by the Romans and probably still fairly common in Anglo-Saxon times around sites of former Roman settlements. Because all three had stinging hairs, were not otherwise strongly differentiated and were equally effective as medicine, they were not separately identified but were all called by the single name *nettle*. So while we can give a Linnaean specific name to *red dead-nettle* because colour is enough to distinguish it from its close relative *white dead-nettle*, we can go no further with *nettle* than to assign it to the genus *Urtica*, leaving the species designation in doubt. For many plants, identification to genus is good enough for the purposes of herbal medicine; and for such plants we cannot expect medieval herbalists to have gone further.

But when only a single species was useful, we may be given enough

---

[18.] Suppliers of seeds and bedding plants still follow the practice of naming plants according to superficial appearances with little or no regard for their place in a taxonomic scheme; for example, the African violet bears only a vague resemblance to the true violet and belongs to an entirely different family of plants. This practice can lead to enormous confusions when one wants to obtain a plant of a specific species.

information to carry our identification to that species. Recent studies in non-Western cultures show that their peoples can match Western botanists and zoologists in assigning plants and animals to groups which correspond remarkably closely to Linnaean classification. This has been shown by Ernst Mayr, working on birds with a Stone Age tribe in Papua New Guinea, and by Brent Berlin, working on plants with the Tzeltal Indians of Mexico. Both groups are able to differentiate birds or plants to the same degree of precision and relationship as a trained scientist using the Linnaean system.[19] When we try to identify plants in the Old English records, we should keep these modern findings in mind, because they imply that pre-Linnaean taxonomies can be remarkably accurate within non-Linnaean frameworks and that if organisms have an important function in a society they may be accurately differentiated or even overdifferentiated by making varietal distinctions within a single species. This we still do with strains of domestic animals and cultivated plants, as is clear from our many names for breeds of dogs and horses and for varieties of apples, for example.

Singer properly drew attention to the dangers inherent in what he called the 'semantics of Anglo-Saxon plant-names'. He wrote: 'Those who have sought to identify plant-names in ancient languages have too often treated the semantics of these words as though they were stable. But they have never been stable.'[20] In this he was absolutely correct. One has only to ask the next person what he means by *daisy* and depending on his background he may describe the true daisy, *Bellis perennis*, or the ox-eye daisy, *Chrysanthemum leucanthemum*, both of which were medicinal herbs, but used for different ailments and given different names by medieval herbalists. So attempts to identify a plant from its Old English name only are usually doomed to failure unless we can show that the name has remained attached to a single species since Anglo-Saxon times, as is true for some cultivated and wild food plants. However, there is another property of plants which has shown remarkable stability for over two thousand years: their use in medicine. I have already shown that the medicinal properties assigned by Aldhelm in the seventh century to the dwarf elder (wallwort), *Sambucus ebulus*, are those given in modern herbals. As a consequence, we have from their uses in medical recipes clues to the identity of herbs

---

[19] These data from Papua New Guinea and Mexico are found together in S. J. Gould, *The Panda's Thumb* (New York, 1982), pp. 204–13 ('A Quahog is a Quahog').

[20] Grattan and Singer, *Anglo-Saxon Magic*, p. 85.

which, taken with any other available clues, including names, may lead to safer identifications than can be obtained from names alone.

How a combination of semantics and medical efficacy may be combined to suggest an identification is shown by OE *ælfþone*, a plant whose identity is beset by many difficulties. Its appearance is nowhere described in the Old English records, nor are glosses of any help. Cockayne's guess that it was enchanter's nightshade, *Circaea lutetiana*, is just that, a guess and a poor one.[21] Modern herbals do not mention it by that name. Nils Thun has recently re-opened the question of identification by pointing out that the second element of the Old English name, -*þone*, is identical with the Old Saxon *thona* which means 'vine', 'creeper'.[22] On this basis and that of German and Dutch plant names in which the first element is *alp-* or *alf-*, and the second an element meaning 'vine' and used to designate the woody nightshade (*Solanum dulcamara*), Thun suggests that there is good reason to suppose that *ælfþone* is the woody nightshade. How does this identification based on semantics stand up to the use of woody nightshade in medicine?

Since the time of the Greek rhizotomists and botanists a group of plants of quite diverse appearances but all belonging to the family Solanaceae – namely henbane (*Hyoscyamus* spp.), thornapple (*Datura* spp.), mandrake (*Mandragora officinarum*), deadly nightshade (*Atropa belladonna*) and black nightshade (*Solanum nigrum*) – all containing the same or related alkaloids of marked potency, have been grouped together; in Northern Europe woody nightshade (*S. dulcamara*) has been associated with them where it also has been used in medicine. The concentration of alkaloids in some of these species depends greatly on the soil in which they are grown and on their exposure to direct sunlight, so that a plant of black nightshade or woody nightshade may be relatively innocuous in one location and pharmacologically active in another. This may explain Aldhelm's attributing to woody nightshade properties more often associated with deadly nightshade. It also increases the difficulty of assigning a modern name to an Old English name in the absence of evidence other than that of the name.

In Old English medicine *ælfþone* was prescribed in nine recipes; three are for *ælfadl*, which seems to have been an eruptive skin condition, two for *micel lic*, which we have seen may have been also some kind of ailment affecting the skin, one was a *leoht drenc* ('light drink', 'tonic'), one a fomentation for *lyftadl* ('paralysis'), one a drink against *deofol* (probably

---

[21] *Leechdoms*, ed. Cockayne II, 368. [22] Thun, 'The Malignant Elves', pp. 378–96.

some form of mental affliction) and one a drink against *weden heorte* (probably 'madness'). A modern herbal has this to say about the medicinal properties of woody nightshade: 'Its action is alterative, and it particularly affects all the organs of the senses. It is very helpful in skin diseases and rheumatism and in bringing relief to paralyzed limbs.'[23] This description of its uses is found in other recent herbals and is in remarkably close agreement with Anglo-Saxon usage. If Thun's analysis of the meaning of the name is correct, *ælfþone* is a vine. Of the group of solanaceous plants considered here, only woody nightshade is a vine. This agreement between semantic and medicinal analyses gives strong support to the inference that OE *ælfþone* and woody nightshade are the same plant.

The identification of *hellebore* in Anglo-Saxon England gives further insight into the problem of medieval plant names. The name is glossed as *wedeberge* ('mad berry') and *þung* ('poisonous plant'). In the older Latin literature *helleborus* was used for plants of two unrelated genera, *Helleborus* and *Veratrum*, neither of which has berries (*berge*), their fruits being dry capsules. Both are poisonous, justifying the name *þung*, and cause violent purging and vomiting. 'Armed with roots of either kind of hellebore, the [physician] could raise blisters, evoke sneezing, vomiting, and diarrhea; induce delirium, muscular cramps, asphyxia; even cause the heart to stop.'[24] A clue to a plant which some Anglo-Saxons took to be *helleborus* is given by Aldhelm in his *Enigma* xcviii, entitled 'Helleborus', where his description of *helleborus* almost certainly refers to the woody nightshade, *Solanum dulcamara*.[25] The symptoms of poisoning he described – including disturbances of the heart, delirium and involuntary, purposeless movements of the limbs – are those to be expected from the ingestion of atropine, an alkaloid in deadly nightshade, *Atropa belladonna*, and in species of *Hyoscyamus* and *Datura*. But ingestion of woody nightshade is said also to cause 'vomiting, vertigo, convulsion, weakened heart, paralysis'.[26] It would seem that there was confusion between the hellebores and species of nightshade because of superficial resemblances between the symptoms of poisoning, and that in some instances, such as Aldhelm's, the name 'hellebore' became attached to the nightshades. It is now impossible,

[23] F. Bianchini and F. Corbetta, *Health Plants of the World* (New York, 1975), p. 142.

[24] Majno, *The Healing Hand*, p. 189.

[25] M. L. Cameron, 'Aldhelm as Naturalist: a Re-Examination of some of his *Enigmata*', *Peritia* 4 (1985), 117–33.

[26] S. Foster and J. A. Duke, *A Field Guide to Medicinal Plants* (Boston, 1990), p. 182.

unless we have information on the appearance of a plant called 'hellebore' by the Anglo-Saxons, to decide which Linnaean group to assign it to.

The Old English *Herbarium* is often useful in determining the identification of Old English plant names, because the translator usually gave an Old English equivalent for each Latin name. But his equations must be used with caution, because he sometimes made mistakes. An interesting error is his translation of *herba gallicrus* by *attorlaþe*, an otherwise unidentified plant name.[27] There is little doubt that *herba gallicrus* in the Latin *Herbarium* is the grass which has been identified as cockspur-grass (*Echinocloa* (*Panicum*) *crus-galli*). Illustrations of the plant in copies of the Latin *Herbarium* show a grass; the illustration in Cotton Vitellius C. iii is of no help as it shows horehound and properly belongs to the following chapter. Only one use for *gallicrus* was given, as an ingredient in a dressing for the bite of dog. *Attorlaþe* is an ingredient of more than thirty remedies in the *Leechbooks* and *Lacnunga*, none of them for animal bites of any kind. How then did the translator come to equate it with *herba gallicrus*?

It appears that he made an identification based on semantics, which failed, as such identifications so often do. Let us try to follow his probable line of reasoning. Not knowing the plant *gallicrus* he took its name literally as meaning 'chicken-leg' or 'chicken-foot'. He knew that Pliny had described a group of medicinal plants which he called *pedes gallinacei* ('chicken-feet'), also known as *capnos* from their Greek name καπνός ('smoke').[28] The translator assumed that Pliny's *pedes gallinacei* were the same plants as he called *attorlaþe*, and translated accordingly. Now, Pliny's plants can be identified with members of the closely related genera *Fumaria* and *Corydalis*, not differentiated by ancient and medieval herbalists but considered by them as a single group. The medical uses assigned to plants of these genera in modern herbals (and by Pliny and Dioscorides[29]) are remarkably similar to those which the Anglo-Saxons assigned to *attorlaþe*, which is confirmed by the close agreement in uses of *attorlaþe* and the *fumitory/corydalis* group of medicinal plants.

Since the time of Cockayne, OE *æþelferðingwyrt* has been equated with stitchwort (*Stellaria holostea*), an identification which has recently been revived.[30] I do not doubt this identification, but I think it is too exclusive.

---

[27] *Herbarium*, ed. de Vriend, pp. 90 and 299.   [28] Pliny, *HN* VII.246–7.

[29] *Dioscurides de Materia Medica*, ed. Wellmann II, 262.

[30] P. Kitson, 'Two Old English Plant Names and Related Matters', *English Studies* 69 (1988), 97–112.

The genus *Stellaria* contains another species, the common chickweed (*S. media*) which has a long history in herbal medicine and which should also be considered as an equivalent to OE *æþelferðingwyrt*, whereas stitchwort is rarely used in medicine except to treat a 'stitch' in the side (hence its name).[31] *Æþelferðingwyrt* was an ingredient in seven prescriptions in the Old English records: four were salves to treat respectively *spring* (an 'abscess' or 'carbuncle'), *dolh* (a 'wound'), a galled place on a horse, and *ða blacan bleagene* ('the black blains'); one was a *holy salve*, purpose not given, but compounded from a host of ingredients with much prayer and ritual; one was a drink for *healsoman* ('inflammation of the throat'); and one a drink for *þeor* (cutaneous conditions associated with vitamin deficiencies). A recent herbal has this to say about chickweed:

> Demulcent, refrigerant. The fresh leaves have been employed as a poultice for inflammation and indolent ulcers with beneficial results. A poultice of Chickweed enclosed in muslin is a sure remedy for a carbuncle or an external abscess. The water in which Chickweed is boiled should also be used to bathe the affected part . . . Chickweed [juice] has also been recommended . . . taken internally for scurvy. The plant chopped and boiled in lard makes a fine green cooling ointment, good for piles and sores, and cutaneous diseases . . . An infusion of the dried herb is efficacious in coughs and hoarseness.[32]

We see that the medical applications of OE *æþelferðingwyrt* and chickweed (*S. media*) are so similar that they are almost certainly the same plant. Since both it and stitchwort (*S. holostea*) are common, it is likely also that either was used depending on which was more readily available. But, given the close agreement between the uses of chickweed and OE *æþelferðingwyrt* compared with the restricted use of stitchwort, it should not be claimed that stitchwort alone represents *æþelferðingwyrt*.

Sometimes it may be impossible to identify a plant by a single Linnaean name because the Anglo-Saxons used a single name for totally unrelated plants. This is the problem with the plant name *brunwyrt* (*brunewyrt*), in which the first element *brun-* may refer to a brown colour or to a disease of the fauces and throat, in Old English *bruneþa* (probably 'diphtheria'). Early herbals describe a disease (in German called *Brune* or *Bräune*) which affected soldiers in camp, causing a darkening of the tongue and lining of the

---

[31] For chickweed, see Grieve, *A Modern Herbal*, pp. 195–6. Stitchwort is not mentioned in recent herbals; the only reference I can find is in Fernie, *Old Fashioned Herbal Remedies*, pp. 490–2, which appears to be a reprint of an undated nineteenth-century publication.

[32] Grieve, *A Modern Herbal*, p. 196.

mouth and throat, and for which the plant prunella ('self-heal', *Prunella vulgaris*) was a specific remedy, the plant getting its name accordingly.[33] But this was not the only plant which was called *brunwyrt*. In the Old English medical records a plant called *brunwyrt* was an ingredient of several recipes for wounds, sore limbs and joints, lung disease, inflammation of the throat, intestinal worms, erysipelatic eruptions and *micel lic* (a cutaneous affliction). Cockayne suggested that more than one species may have been called *brunwyrt*; he suggested asplenium (*Ceterach officinarum*); figwort (*Scrophularia nodosa* and *S. aquatica*) and self-heal (*Prunella vulgaris*).[34] The name appears in three Durham glosses: *Radiolum eofer-fearn vel brun-vyrt*; *Splenion brunvyrt*; *Vaccinium brunvyrt*.[35] Similarly, in the Old English *Herbarium*, *brunewyrt* translates Latin *splenion*.[36] It has also been suggested that it may be betony (*Stachys betonica*). This last identification is most unlikely, because *brunwyrt* and *betonica* are prescribed together in four Old English recipes. As for the Durham glosses, *radiolus* (*-um*) is elsewhere glossed by words referring to the ribs or radius bone of the forearm. Referred to a fern it could be used to describe the frond of the *eofer-fearn* ('boar fern', *Polypodium vulgare*) which is not unlike a ribcage in appearance. I have no idea what *vaccinium* meant, except that it could have had nothing to do with the modern genus *Vaccinium*.

A common feature of the plants suggested for OE *brunwyrt* is that they all have some suggestion of brown about them. The backs of the fronds of spleenwort (*Asplenium*) are covered with brown scales, the flowers of figwort are brownish purple, the bracts of the flowering and fruiting head of self-heal are distinctly brown. Thus it seems likely that to the Anglo-Saxons the *brun-* of OE *brunwyrt* may have meant brown, although it may also have referred to a disease of the mouth and throat, and this gives us a clue to its appearance. Spleenwort is prescribed for only one ailment in the Latin *Herbarium*, namely enlargement of the spleen. Apart from the reference in the *Herbarium*, *brunwyrt* does not seem to have had this function in Anglo-Saxon medicine. Figwort and self-heal are vulneraries and used for skin eruptions.

[Figwort] has been called the Scrofula Plant, on account of its value in all cutaneous eruptions, abscesses, wounds, etc. . . . . A decoction of it is made for

---

[33] See, for example, Gerard, *The Herball*, p. 634. See also *Leechdoms*, ed. Cockayne II, 373, s.v. *bruneþan*.

[34] *Leechdoms*, ed. Cockayne II, 374.

[35] Von Lindheim, 'Das Durhamer Pflanzenglossar', pp. 1–81.

[36] *Herbarium*, ed. de Vriend, p. 100.

external use, and the fresh leaves are also made into an ointment . . . It has diuretic and anodyne properties . . . This species [*Scrophularia nodosa*] is most employed, principally as a fomentation for sprains, swellings, inflammations, wounds and diseased parts, especially in scrofulous sores and gangrene.[37]

It gets the name figwort from its use to treat 'the fig' or haemorrhoids. It contains cardio-active glycosides which make its ingestion unsafe except under a physician's supervison.

[Self-heal is] astringent, styptic and tonic. Self-Heal is still in use in modern herbal treatment as a useful astringent for inward and outward use. An infusion of the herb . . . taken in doses of a wineglassful, is considered a general strengthener. Sweetened with honey, it is good for a sore and relaxed throat or ulcerated mouth, for both of which purposes it also makes a good gargle. For internal bleeding and for piles, the infusion is also used as an injection.[38]

Culpeper recommended it as especially good for 'inward and outward wounds, outwardly in unguents and plasters for outward . . . for inward wounds or ulcers in the body, for bruises or falls and hurts . . . It is an especial remedy for all green wounds to close the lips of them.'[39]

It appears that for the ailments for which *brunwyrt* was prescribed in the Old English remedies, either figwort or self-heal would have been satisfactory, but that spleenwort would have been of no use. Where tonics or potions were to be swallowed, it would have been unsafe to administer figwort except in small doses, whereas self-heal was safe. It is most probable that both plants went by the name of *brunwyrt*, at different times and places, so that today we are only able to conclude that *brunwyrt* may have been *Prunella vulgaris* or *Scrophularia nodosa* (or at times *S. aquatica*) or all three, but that it was not betony (*Stachys betonica*) or spleenwort (*Ceterach officinarum*) or any other fern, except by mistaken analogy (as in the Durham gloss). That the OE name *brunwyrt* was used for the figworts is supported by the translation of *splenion* by *brunwyrt* in the *Herbarium*, because the leaves and stem of *Scrophularia aquatica* bear some resemblance to the fronds of spleenwort; accordingly, the translator, who knew figwort as *brunwyrt*, may well have assumed that the plant illustrated in his exemplar was the same one. On the other hand, the illustration in the Old

---

[37] Grieve, *A Modern Herbal*, p. 313.   [38] *Ibid.*, p. 732.

[39] N. Culpeper, *The English Physician Enlarged* (London, 1799), pp. 278–9. There are also countless modern editions, many incomplete: a reliable one is *Culpeper's Complete Herbal* (London, [n.d.]).

English version looks more like self-heal, as if to the illustrator that is what *brunwyrt* meant.[40] It seems that the Anglo-Saxons could be as confused by their plant names as we are.

These examples of efforts to identify plants in Old English texts show how difficult the task can be, and equally how doubtful the results may be. It appears that even in Anglo-Saxon times different plants were given the same or similar names at different times and in different places, so that the Anglo-Saxons themselves seem to have been sometimes confused in their identification. Their confusion may not often have been serious, because the plants confused often had the same medical uses and efficacies. There was also a tendency to give a single name to a group of closely related plants having the same medical properties, as seems to have been true for OE *attorlathe* signifying plants of the two genera *Fumaria* and *Corydalis*, although it must be noted that some recipes specify the 'greater' *attorlathe* or the 'lesser' *attorlathe*, indicating that differences were recognized in spite of a common name. It is safe to say that where exact differentiation was useful or necessary it was made, but where plants of similar appearance had the same medical properties they were given a single name, even if to a modern botanist they should be distinguished from one another. All this makes it difficult and often impossible to give to a single Old English plant name a modern Linnaean designation. For the purposes of herbal medicine, however, single-species identification is not always necessary.

Of the two questions asked at the beginning of this chapter we have been able to give a qualified answer to the first one, 'What substances were prescribed in remedies?' by showing that animal and mineral products are not difficult to identify and that most plants can be identified to the same degree that they were identified by the Anglo-Saxons and other herbalists of their time, but that a number remain whose identity is doubtful or which cannot be identified at all. To the second question, 'Were these substances obtainable in England at that time?' the answer is 'Yes, a substance called for in a recipe was almost certain to be obtainable, whether it was available to all physicians at all times or only on occasion and in certain places.' It now remains to look at the third question, 'What was the therapeutic value of these substances; could they be expected to have beneficial effects on the ailments for which they were prescribed?' For an answer we turn to the next chapter.

[40] London, BL, Cotton Vitellius C. iii, 38r.

12

Rational medicine

At the end of the last chapter we asked: 'What was the therapeutic value of these substances; could they be expected to have beneficial effects on the ailments for which they were prescribed?' The answer has usually been: 'No'. Charles Singer put it emphatically:

In the Early English medical documents there is no mention of the physiological action of drugs. There is no trace in them of any knowledge of anatomy or physiology . . . To estimate the therapeutic armoury of the leech it would be necessary to enumerate all the plant names in all the texts. The result of so tiresome a task would not repay the effort. [1]

His pupil, Wilfrid Bonser, was equally emphatic: 'One must not necessarily look in a prescription for any physiological effect which the ingredients might have had on a patient.'[2] In another context he wrote: 'Sterile formulas, which could be applied without any exercise of reasoning, alone survived for use during the Dark Ages. It is these, therefore, with very few exceptions, which appear in Anglo-Saxon medical practice.'[3]

If we rephrase our question more specifically: 'Did ancient and medieval physicians use ingredients and methods which were likely to have had beneficial effects on the patients whose ailments they treated?', then I think the answer is 'Yes, and their prescriptions were about as good as anything prescribed before the mid-twentieth century'.

As we have seen, most Anglo-Saxon remedies were of plant origin. Even today, at least one-quarter of the drugs used in medicine are from flowering plants, or prepared synthetically to copy plant products. Many of the

[1] Grattan and Singer, *Anglo-Saxon Magic*, p. 92.
[2] Bonser, *Medical Background*, p. 8.
[3] *Ibid.*, p. 35.

plants supplying drugs today were in use in ancient times as well. This implies that some ancient remedies must have contained beneficial substances. Much evaluation of plants for their medicinal value is now in progress in pharmaceutical laboratories and the results are often of much interest. The greater part of the identifiable ingredients of the Anglo-Saxon pharmacopoeia are still to be found in herbal collections and are used for the same purposes, so that we may say that Anglo-Saxon remedies were probably as good as those recommended by herbalists today. Moreover, a surprisingly large number of their ingredients are known from recent investigation to contain substances of real therapeutic value and to have been used by them for conditions where their therapeutic value should have had beneficial effects. These medicines certainly did not have the marvellous efficacy of modern antibiotics and chemotherapeutic drugs, but they do seem to have been just as good as anything available up to the end of the nineteenth century, and to have been applied with much the same appreciation of their therapeutic values.

Lewis Thomas in an autobiographical sketch tells how his father treated his patients in his general practice in the early years of the twentieth century. He used the standard medicines which had been the stock-in-trade of all medical practitioners for hundreds of years, but had no real knowledge of their medical effectiveness and thought of many of them as placebos which, doing no harm, gave the patient the feeling that something was being done for him while the illness ran through its normal course. Yet this man was an able physician with a record of success in treating his patients.[4]

In spite of this gloomy appraisal of general medicine before the present century, there were medicines which were of some help to patients. No doubt their efficacy was not all that great, but they continued in use up to our own day, and we may now look at a sampling of them from the *Leechbooks* and *Lacnunga* to examine their usefulness. For example, for millennia copper has been used to prevent and to treat bacterial infections; its salts are cytotoxic, killing all living cells, but the amount of poisoning one would receive from the application of a copper salt to an infected wound would be small compared with the benefit from its killing of the bacteria in the wound. The earliest example of a recipe for infection that I have seen is an Assyrian prescription reported by Campbell Thompson: 'If his flesh has poison and lassitude, and shrinking of the flesh . . . [here

[4] L. Thomas, *The Youngest Science: Notes of a Medicine-Watcher* (New York, 1983), p. 15.

follows a long list of plants and plant products] . . . thou shalt put, boil in a small copper pan, wash him therewith.'[5] In this recipe, probably the most effective antibacterial agent was the copper salt produced in the pan when the acidic plant materials were cooked. Anyone familiar with Ancient Egyptian paintings knows the green pigment around the eyes. This eye-paint was made from ores of copper and was in origin a prophylactic against infection of the eyes. Where copper ores were not readily available, as in Greece and Asia Minor, copper acetate was made by putting vinegar in a pot, covering the pot with a brass or copper lid and leaving it for a few days, or by hanging a brass or copper sheet above vinegar in a closed vessel.[6]

An outstanding example of a remedy likely to have been helpful is this one from Bald's *Leechbook*:

Make an eye salve for a stye: take *cropleac* 'onion' and garlic equal amounts of both, pound well together, take wine and bull's gall equal amounts of both, mix with the 'leeks', then put in a brass vessel, let stand for nine nights in the brass vessel, strain through a cloth and clear well, put in a horn and about night time put on the eye with a feather; the best remedy.[7]

A staphylococcal infection of a hair follicle is the usual cause of a stye on the eyelid. The ingredients of the salve were onion, garlic, bull's gall, wine and copper salts formed in the brass vessel. Onion and garlic are antibiotics, garlic juice in particular, even at high dilution, inhibiting the growth of species of *staphylococcus* and of various other kinds of bacteria.[8] Bull's gall, which is still in the pharmacopoeia as oxgall, has detergent properties which make it effective against Gram-positive bacteria such as the *staphylococci*.[9] Medieval wine would have contained a generous amount of acetic acid as well as the tartarates resulting from fermentation. These would react with the copper of the brass vessel to form copper salts (acetates

---

[5] R. C. Thompson, 'Assyrian Prescriptions for Treating Bruises or Swellings', *American Journal of Semitic Languages and Literatures* 47 (1930), 1–25.

[6] *Dioscuridis de Materia Medica*, ed. Wellmann III, 49.

[7] *Leechdoms*, ed. Cockayne II, 34: 'Wyrc eagsealfe wiþ wænne: genim cropleac 7 garleac begea emfela, gecnuwa wel tosomne, genim win 7 fearres geallan begea emfela, gemeng wiþ þy leace, do þonne on arfæt, læt standan nigon niht on þæm arfæt, awring þurh claþ 7 gehlyttre wel, do on horn 7 ymb niht do mid feþere on eage; se betsta læcedom.'

[8] E. Block, 'The Chemistry of Garlic and Onions', *Scientific American* 252.3 (1985), 114–19.

[9] Dr R. Brown, personal communication.

and tartarates), as would also any acids in the plant juices. These salts are all cytotoxic, destroying all living cells, including bacteria.[10] There would be loss of some tissue cells, but that would be a small price to pay for the destruction of many bacteria and the clearing up of the infection. It is important to notice that the preparation was kept in the brass vessel for only nine days, after which it was strained and the clear liquid stored in a non-reactive horn container until needed.

Here was a remedy containing four antibiotic agents, three of them, onion, garlic and gall, especially active against Gram-positive bacteria such as the *staphylococci* most likely to have caused a stye, and copper salts toxic to all cells. Applied to a stye, this medicine should have helped to destroy bacteria at the site of infection and inhibit the spread of infection to other sites. It was proper to call it *se betsta læcedom*. No source or analogue has been found; it would be interesting to know how and where it was developed.

A number of other remedies for the eyes in Bald's *Leechbook* also prescribe copper salts as one ingredient.[11] Dioscorides recommended onion and garlic for infections including those of the eyes,[12] and also bull's gall.[13] We must bear in mind that this was all done when there was no knowledge of bacterial pathogens.[14] Yet the composition of the medicine implies a long line of observant physicians who developed a treatment specific for the causative agent with no knowledge of bacteria. It was adamantly not a sterile formula, devoid of reasoning.

That copper salts were known to be beneficial in treating infections is clear from the number of remedies in which they were an ingredient. That physicians did recognize their worth is also clear in the last recipe of the second chapter of Bald's *Leechbook*, where curds (containing lactic acid) are to be added to the dregs in a copper vessel from which another medicine had been drained. The last injunction to the user is: 'Then scrape out the vessel, that will be a good salve for those who have thick (i.e., swollen, infected) eyelids.'[15]

[10] Majno, *The Healing Hand*, pp. 186–8.   [11] *Leechdoms*, ed. Cockayne II, 38.

[12] *Dioscuridis de Materia Medica*, ed. Wellmann II, 217–19.   [13] *Ibid.*, pp. 159–60.

[14] The long folk history of the onion as a bactericide is not yet over; I remember that when I was a child (about seventy years ago) my grandmother kept a syrup of onions in honey or sugar to be taken for a sore throat (usually caused by another Gram-positive bacterium, a *streptococcus*), and that our family doctor thought of the cure as pure superstition. He offered nothing in its place, however.

[15] *Leechdoms*, ed. Cockayne II, 38: 'Screp þonne of þæm fæte þæt biþ swiðe god sealf þam men þe hæfð þicca bræwes.'

Another remedy for the eyes shows the development of a recipe through time and the care with which its compounding might be carried out. It is found in two very similar forms in Bald's *Leechbook* and has been quoted already in ch. 10; I shall repeat it here in order to analyse it: 'Medicines for dimness of the eyes: take the juice or blossoms of celandine, mix with bumblebees' honey, put in a brass vessel, make lukewarm skilfully over warm coals until it is cooked. This is a good medicine for dimness of the eyes.'[16] Here again we find copper salts in a remedy for infected eyes. We have seen in ch. 10 that it has sources/analogues in the *Herbarium*, Pliny and Dioscorides. In those sources, Attic honey was specified. The word *atticus* ('from Attica') early became confused with *attacus* (an insect, perhaps some kind of locust), and both then came to be used to describe a wild bee.[17] As the bumblebee is the only wild bee in England which stores enough honey to make it worthwhile to rob its nests, the Latin *atticus* came to mean the same as *dora*, the 'bumblebee'. Celandine is the greater celandine (*Chelidonium majus*); it exudes a bright orange latex from all injured parts. This latex in the fresh state is powerfully irritant, but after drying or heating, the irritant property is much reduced or destroyed. In this state it has been used successfully since time immemorial to remove films or spots from the cornea of the eye.[18] Copper salts and honey are bactericidal. The remedy may have been of some help for a bacterial infection of the eye complicated by spotting or filming of the cornea. But why the warning in the Old English recipe about warming the preparation 'skilfully'? Honey and celandine juice are both rather thick liquids and so burn easily when heated. This explains the need for a gentle fire and for extreme care in the cooking. Someone along the way in the preparation of this recipe thought it important to give warning of these problems.

Not understanding the rationale behind this remedy, Storms treated it as a magical one: 'The use of bumble-bee honey, of a brass vessel, and the heating over glowing coals instead of over an ordinary fire, together with the adverb *listum*, "skilfully, cunningly" belong to the sphere of magic.'[19]

---

[16] *Ibid.*: 'Læcedomas wiþ eagna miste: genim celeþenian seaw oþþe blostman, gemeng wið dorena hunig, gedo on ærenfæt, wlece listum on wearmum gledum oþþæt hit gesoden sie. Þis bið god læcedom wiþ eagna dimnesse.'

[17] *Herbarium*, ed. de Vriend, p. 332 (n. to M IV.13) has a discussion of the confusion between *attacus* and *atticus*, etc., together with references to the pertinent literature.

[18] Grieve, *A Modern Herbal*, pp. 178–9.

[19] Storms, *Anglo-Saxon Magic*, pp. 133–4.

He also thought that the remedy for a stye was magic because of the use of a copper vessel.[20] But these two examples should warn us that not all remedies in Anglo-Saxon collections were based on simple superstition, but that some of them, at least, were the result of long and patient observation of the effects of various medicines, and that we must not accept unthinkingly Bonser's remark: 'Sterile formulas, which could be applied without any exercise of reasoning, alone survived for use during the Dark Ages.'[21]

So long as that kind of opinion of the 'Dark Ages' persists, even rationally conceived remedies tend to be thought magical. In *Lacnunga* there is a treatment which reads: 'For a swelling, take root of lily and shoot of elder and leaf of porleek [most likely 'leek' and certainly some kind of onion] and shred very small and pound thoroughly and put on a thick cloth and bind on.'[22] Storms thought this was a charm because 'the three ingredients of which the paste consists show some thickening or swelling, and just as these swellings disappear by cutting them up and pounding them, so the swelling of the patient will disappear.'[23] But a modern herbalist, Mrs Grieve, had different opinions of the value of these plants used as in the recipe:

Owing to their highly mucilaginous properties, the bulbs [of the lily] are chiefly employed externally, boiled in milk or water, as emollient cataplasms for tumours, ulcers and external inflammations, and have been much used for this purpose in popular practice. The fresh bulb, bruised and applied to hard tumours, softens and ripens them sooner than any other applications.[24]

The same herbalist wrote of the dwarf elder: 'The leaves, bruised and laid on boils and scalds, have a healing effect.'[25] She did not write anything about the leek, but wrote of garlic: 'It is sometimes externally applied . . . to disperse hard swellings.'[26] Considering that members of the onion genus share most of their properties, differing most in the quantity of constituents rather than in having different ones, one may guess that leek would have the same effect as garlic but to a lesser degree. There can be little

---

[20] *Ibid.*, pp. 71–2.   [21] Bonser, *Medical Background*, p. 8.

[22] Grattan and Singer, *Anglo-Saxon Magic*, p. 106: 'Wið geswel, genim lilian moran 7 ellenes spryttinge 7 porleaces leaf 7 scearfa swiðe smale 7 cnuca swiðe 7 do on ðicne claþ 7 bind on.'

[23] Storms, *Anglo-Saxon Magic*, p. 29.   [24] Grieve, *A Modern Herbal*, p. 483.

[25] *Ibid.*, p. 277.

[26] *Ibid.*, p. 344.

doubt, therefore, that the three ingredients of this remedy were used for their known therapeutic value, not because of their magic shapes.

Until the late nineteenth century most medicines were of plant origin. After Pasteur and Lister had demonstrated the involvement of 'germs' in many diseases and septic conditions, there was a revolution in medical practice, one result of which was the introduction of new drugs, many of them of chemical origin, and a rejection of the old herbal cures. At the same time the application to medicine of the scientific method of controlled experiments opened up new fields and understanding of disease and health, and prompted medical researchers to reject the old medicine on the grounds that no experimental or observational discoveries of medical value could have been made prior to the use of their method. In more recent times there has been a return to investigation of the therapeutic properties of herbs with interesting results which illuminate their use by ancient and medieval practitioners. We have seen an example of this in the remedy for a stye; it is recent work on the detergent properties of gall and the antiseptic properties of the onion genus which has shown the value of that medicine. We can find similar, if less spectacular, instances in the use of other plants as medicine.

In the old medicine, various plantains (*Plantago* spp.) were frequently prescribed for various ailments. They were a common ingredient of applications for wounds and for certain skin conditions. They appear in a few magical recipes; plantain was invoked in the Old English *Nine Herbs Charm* in terms which seem to imply some knowledge of its antibacterial properties: 'So may you withstand venom and infection, and the loathsome thing which roams through the land',[27] where the reference seems to be to what we would now call bacterial infections. Recent work has shown that the plantains contain aucubin, a potent antibiotic, in all their parts, especially plentiful in *Plantago major* (the common broad-leaved plantain), *P. lanceolata* (ribwort) and *P. media* (hoary plantain). Aucubin is a glucoside which is itself inactive; in the presence of a suitable enzyme such as emulsin (a β-glucosidase found in the plantains and made available when they are crushed) it is hydrolysed to an active aglycone form. Thus, any part of a ground-up plantain will show antibiotic activity against *staphylococci*, *streptococci* and *clostridia* (the bacteria responsible for skin infections, for throat and mouth infections and for tetanus respectively). 'Against a

---

[27] Grattan and Singer, *Anglo-Saxon Magic*, p. 152: 'Swa þu wiðstonde attre 7 onflyge/ 7 þæm laþan þe geond lond fereð.'

culture of *Staphylococcus aureus*, 1 ml of 2% aqueous solution of aucubin had in the presence of β-glucosidase the same effect as 600 I.U. penicillin.'[28] The crushed plant must be freshly prepared, because the activated form of aucubin is highly unstable and soon loses its activity. Given the long-continued use of freshly crushed plantain to treat wounds one may infer that it did exert observably beneficial effects and that its activity against *attre 7 onflyge* was appreciated.

Were these requirements of freshly crushed plant material followed in Anglo-Saxon treatments for wounds? Here is a selection of remedies from Bald's *Leechbook*: 'For sore feet or swelling from much walking, plantain pounded and mixed with vinegar.' 'If it [a boil] is in the ear, beat plantain and feverfew and pepper, strain into the ear.' 'Here are wound salves for all wounds . . . plantain beaten, mixed with old lard (fresh is no good).' 'A wound salve: take plantain seed, grind small, spread on the wound; it will soon be better.' 'For a wound by a dog . . . plantain, beat, lay on . . . Again, take plantain root, pound with lard, put on the wound; then it will clear away the poison.'[29] Of the forty-eight remedies containing plantain in the three *Leechbooks*, twenty-five are for conditions where its antibiotic properties would have been of benefit. There can be no doubt that plantain was used for its known effectiveness for wounds and infections. Of the remedies in the *Leechbooks*, only three are not paralleled in modern herbal medicine.

In the *Leechbooks* there are some half-dozen remedies for wounds and for *lungen adl* ('lung disease') in which lichen is an ingredient. The sources of the lichens were specified as a hazel tree, a sloethorn tree, a birch tree, a church, a crucifix and a hallowed crucifix. Churches and crucifixes suggest magical properties in ingredients taken from them. But let us look at some of these recipes. 'Wound salve: hazel lichen and the lower part of holly rind and githrife, pound the herbs very well, mix with butter, cook

---

[28] O. Sticher, 'Plant Mono-, Di- and Sesquiterpenoids with Pharmacological or Therapeutic Activity', in *New Natural Products and Plant Drugs with Pharmacological, Biological or Therapeutic Activity*, ed. H. Wagner and P. Wolff (Berlin, 1976), p. 149.

[29] *Leechdoms*, ed. Cockayne II, 68: 'Wið fota sare oþþe geswelle fram miclum gange, wegbræde getrifulad 7 wið eced gemenged.'; 80: 'Gif he [spring] on earan sie, gebeate wegbrædan 7 feferfugean 7 pipor, wring on þæt eare.'; 90: 'Her sindon dolhsealfa to eallum wundum . . . wegbræde gebeaten wið ealdne rysele gemenged (fersc ne nyt bið).'; 90: 'Dolhsealf, genim wegbrædan sæd, getrifula smale, scead on þa wunde, sona bið selre.'; 144: 'Wiþ hundes dolge . . . wegbrædan, gebeat, lege on . . . Eft, genim wegbrædan moran, gecnua wiþ rysle, do on þæt dolh; þonne ascrypð hio þæt ater aweg.'

thoroughly, skim off the foam, strain through a cloth very clean.'[30] 'For spider bite: take *aeferth* the lower part and sloethorn lichen, dry to powder, moisten with honey, dress the wound with it.'[31] 'For lung disease make a salve in butter and eat in milk: take brownwort, meadowwort, birch lichen, catmint, garclife.'[32]

Several common species of lichen or extracts from them are still used in folk and patent medicines, particularly in Scandinavia and Finland. They have constituents which possess antibiotic activity, particularly against *staphylococci* and tubercle bacilli (*Mycobacterium tuberculosis*), so that their use by the Anglo-Saxons for wounds and animal bites and for lung disease seems appropriate. The third recipe quoted above is of particular interest because the medicine was to be boiled in milk. Today Iceland moss (*Cetraria islandica*) and species of *Cladonia* are boiled in milk and the lichen-milk drunk to treat cough and pulmonary tuberculosis.[33] It appears that Anglo-Saxon physicians recognized the therapeutic value of lichens. That the recipes specified the sources from which they were to be gathered may not be a result of superstitious beliefs; lichens are neither easy to describe clearly nor to identify accurately and may have been identified for medicinal purposes by the substrates on which they grew.

Rue is another plant of known medicinal effect; it is a source of rutin, a flavonoid related to hesperidin and quercitrin, which is used as a capillary antihaemorrhagic and corrective of capillary permeability, being useful in cerebrovascular and cardiovascular diseases and other conditions where capillary fragility is a factor.[34] The leaves are very bitter but if chewed are said to leave a refreshing taste in the mouth and to relieve various nervous conditions; they have glands containing a strongly irritant oil which acts as a rubefacient.[35] Rue is an ingredient in thirty-six remedies in the *Leechbooks*: of these about two-thirds are prescribed for ailments for which

---

[30] *Ibid.*, p. 96: 'Dolhsealf: hæsles ragu 7 holen rinde niþewearde 7 gyþrifen, gecnua swiðe wel þa wyrta, gemeng wið buteran, seoð swiðe, fleot of þæt fam, aseoh þur clað swiþe clæne.'

[31] *Ibid.*, pp. 142–4: 'Wiþ gongelwæfran bite nim æferþan niþowearde 7 slahþorn rage, adrig to duste, geþæn mid hunige, lecna þæt dolh mid.'

[32] *Ibid.*, p. 266: 'Wiþ lungen adle wyrc sealfe on buteran 7 þige on meolcum: nim brunewyrt, meodowyrt, berc rago, nefte, garclife.'

[33] K. O. Bartia, 'Antibiotics in Lichens', *The Lichens*, ed. V. Ahmadjian and M. E. Hale (New York and London, 1973), pp. 547–61; Y. Asahina and S. Shibata, *Chemistry of Lichen Substances* (Amsterdam, 1971), pp. 216–24.

[34] Claus and Tylor, *Pharmacognosy*, pp. 145–7.   [35] Grieve, *A Modern Herbal* p. 696.

rue is still recommended in modern herbals. A remedy in *Leechbook III* combines the antibacterial properties of plantain with the antihaemorrhagic properties of rue: 'For a bite by a dog: pound ribwort plantain, lay on the wound, and boil rue in butter; treat the wound with it.'[36]

Henbane is well known for its action in blocking the nerve fibres of the parasympathetic nervous system, and contains also scopolamine which is a hypnotic, inducing a sleep very similar to the natural one.[37] It is an ingredient of thirteen remedies, of which ten are for conditions for which these properties would be important. Pennyroyal is best known as a carminative of use against flatulence and nausea, but it also has antispasmodic properties and causes reflex movements of the uterus.[38] Of seventeen remedies containing pennyroyal twelve are for ailments for which these properties would be useful.

Under the floor of the valetudinarium at Corbridge near Hadrian's Wall archaeologists found a chest filled with scrap iron and brass, presumably to be used to treat wounds in the hospital.[39] Pliny gave a treatment for dysentery which was then often thought to be a wound of the intestines: 'For many disorders, but especially for those suffering from dysentery, water is heated with red-hot iron'.[40] Bald's *Leechbook* has a similar treatment: 'For broken-out inwards: coriander seed well ground up and a little salt, put in sharp wine, put in and heat with a glowing hot iron, give to drink'.[41] Although the value of iron salts for restoring the iron balance of the body is well attested, their use and that of iron rust to treat wounds has not been tested recently, but there is no doubt that they were believed to be effective in promoting healing.

Although iron has played an important magical role in ancient and medieval medicine, it also entered into rational remedies. We have already seen in ch. 2 how enlargement of the spleen and loss of iron from the body

---

[36] *Leechdoms*, ed. Cockayne II, 328: 'Wiþ hundes slite cnuwa ribban, lege on þæt dolh 7 rudan wyl on buteran, lacna mid þæt dolh.'

[37] Claus and Tylor, *Pharmacognosy*, pp. 278–83.

[38] Grieve, *A Modern Herbal*, p. 626.

[39] R. W. Davies, 'A Note on the Hoard of Roman Equipment Buried at Corbridge', *Durham University Journal* 31 (1970), 177–80.

[40] Pliny, *HN* IX.236: 'Calfit etiam ferro candente potus in multis vitiis, privatim vero dysentericis.'

[41] *Leechdoms*, ed. Cockayne II, 236: 'Wiþ tobrocenum innoþum: cellendres sæd wel gegniden 7 lytel sealtes, gedo on scearp win, gedo on 7 gewyrme mid hate glowende isene, sele drincan.'

as a consequence of malaria were treated by a potion containing iron acetate.

Examples from simpler recipes may be more convincing concerning the essential rationality of Anglo-Saxon medicine. I shall draw them from *Leechbook III*, it being the least influenced by Mediterranean culture. Horehound (*Marrubium vulgare*) is still prescribed in lozenges to control an annoying cough. Honey is also used for the same purpose. Two recipes for cough medicines are given together in this *Leechbook*; they have analogues in Marcellus, but are unlikely to be borrowed from him.[42] They read: 'For cough boil a good deal of horehound in water, sweeten a little, give a cupful to drink. Again: horehound, boil strongly in honey, add a little butter, give three or four slices to eat, after the night's fast sup a cupful of the preceding warm drink with it.'[43] The second of these recipes is particularly interesting; it combines the spasmolytic effects of horehound with the antiseptic properties of honey and the soothing effect of butter. This relatively solid mixture melted in the mouth while the warm horehound drink was being supped.

A remedy for bloated stomach or intestines[44] improved on a *Herbarium* recipe[45] by adding garlic mustard (*Alliaria petiolata*) to a decoction of pennyroyal (*Mentha pulegium*). Pennyroyal has well-known carminative properties, but garlic mustard supplies deobstruent and digestive ones as well to make a medicine of wider scope. Similarly, in a remedy for bladder complaint, garlic mustard, which also has diuretic properties was added to a decoction in ale of parsley, whose diuretic properties made it a standard ingredient in medicines for ailments of the bladder.[46] The remaining examples are without analogues and so most probably represent native Anglo-Saxon practices. For diarrhoea cinquefoil (*Potentilla* spp.), which acts powerfully against diarrhoea, and brooklime (*Veronica beccabunga*),

---

[42] *Marcelli De Medicamentis*, ed. Niedermann, pp. 276 and 282.

[43] *Leechdoms*, ed. Cockayne II, 312: 'Wiþ hwostan wyl marubian on wætre godne dæl, geswet hwon, sele drincan scencful. Eft: marbuian, swiðe wyl on hunige, do hwon buteran on, sele III sneda oþþe IIII etan, on neahtnestig besup scencfulne mid wearmes þæs ærran drences.'

[44] *Ibid.*, p. 318: 'Wiþ aþundenesse 7 [gif] men nelle myltan his mete, wyl on wætere polleian 7 leaccersan, sele drincan, him biþ sona sel.'

[45] *Herbarium*, ed de Vriend, p. 140: 'Ad stomachi inflationem aut intestinorum. Herbam puleium ex aqua calida contritum vel ex vino aut per se dato, remitteris cito.'

[46] *Leechdoms*, ed. Cockayne II, 320: 'Wiþ blædder wærce: wudumerce 7 leaccerse, wyl swiþe on ealað, sele drincan.'

which contains much tannin, were boiled in milk with two other herbs of attested value for diarrhoea to make a drink to be taken morning and evening.[47] For intestinal worms this treatment is given: 'If there are worms in one's insides boil green rue in butter, drink a cupful after the night's fast; they will all go away with the stool and he will soon be well.[48] Rue (*Ruta graveolens*) is an effective antihelminthic, although side effects of its ingestion do not recommend it today for this purpose. For a burn, woodruff (*Asperula odorata*) and brooklime (*Veronica beccabunga*), both rich in tannin, were applied in butter with lily (*Lilium candidum*), demulcent and astringent and said to remove pain and inflammation from burns, healing them without scars.[49] A treatment for swollen stomach (or abdomen) was rue, eaten and drunk; rue is a stomachic and the rutin it contains aids in the capillary function of assimilation.[50] Jaundice was treated with dill, coriander and sage boiled in beer until thick and green and drunk after eating a slice of elecampane root cut up in honey; I do not know of any effect of elecampane on the liver, but it and dill and coriander are carminative and sage is recommended for biliousness and liver complaints.[51] Finally, 'If a man's insides be out, pound comfrey, wring through a cloth into milk warm from the cow, wet your hand in it and replace the insides into the man, sew up with silk, then boil comfrey for him nine mornings, unless he have need for it longer.'[52] Comfrey (*Symphytum officinale*) contains allantoin, which is now used topically in

---

[47] *Ibid.*, p. 320.

[48] *Ibid.*, pp. 320–2: 'Gif wyrmas beoþ on mannes innoðe wyl on buteran grene rudan, drinc on neahtnestig scencfulne; hi gewitað ealle aweg mid þy utgange 7 he bið sona hal.'

[49] *Ibid.*, p. 324.

[50] *Ibid.*, p. 356: 'Wiþ magan wærce: rudan sæd 7 cwicseolfor 7 eced, bergen on neahtnestig' ('For stomach trouble: rue seed and quicksilver and vinegar, eat fasting'). The recipe is from *Herbarium*, ed. de Vriend, p. 135: 'Ad stomachi dolorem. Herbae rutae semen cum sulfure vivo et aceto ieiunus gustato.' Note the error in translation which substituted mercury for sulphur; one hopes the recipe was not used in this form.

[51] *Ibid.*, p. 358: 'Eft: dile, celendre, saluian mæst, wyl on swiþum beore þæt hit sie þicce and grene, nim niþewearde eolenan, gesniþ on hunig, ete swa manige snæda swa he mæge; gedrince þæs drences scenc fulne æfter' ('Again: dill, coriander, mast of sage, boil in strong beer so that it may be thick and green; take the lower part of elecampane, slice into honey, let him eat as many slices as he can, let him drink afterwards a cupful of the potion').

[52] *Ibid.*: 'Gif men sie innelfe ute gecnua galluc, awring þurh claið on cuwearme meolce, wæt þine handa þær on 7 gedo þæt innelfe on þone man, geseowe mid seolce, whyl him þonne galluc viii morgnas butan him leng þearf sie.'

suppurating wounds and ulcers to accelerate cell proliferation; it was a wound healer of choice in ancient and medieval times. Whatever one may think of fresh milk as a vehicle for bacterial infection, the intent of the recipe was obviously to supply needed moisture to the protruding intestines and to supply them and the wound with a proven healing ingredient.

It would be easy to continue with analyses of this sort for other medicines, but it is not necessary. It is clear that the Anglo-Saxons prescribed ingredients which should have been of benefit and are still recommended for the same ailments. It is also clear that they recognized the medical properties of many substances and made prescriptions based on these recognitions; not all medieval medicine consisted of 'sterile formulas, which could be applied without any exercise of reasoning',[53] nor is it true that 'one must not necessarily look in a prescription for any physiological effect which the ingredients might have had on a patient.'[54]

I think I have given enough examples to show that their medicines, even when not influenced by more advanced Mediterranean practices, were often rationally conceived and should have contributed to the well-being of the patient. Given the lack of knowledge of physiology and the action of drugs, physicians could choose useful remedies only through long and careful observation. It is because of the observational pragmatism of ancient and medieval practitioners that so many of their medicines were specific for the maladies to which they were applied.

By no means all Anglo-Saxon medicine was rationally conceived. Much of the *materia medica* was magical in intent, magical remedies being used most often to treat ailments intractable to rational medicines, ones which even today do not yield readily to rational procedures. But although magic and superstition played a part in the practice of Anglo-Saxon medicine, it would be wrong to claim that it was the chief part. A careful examination of the Old English texts shows that, while the magical element is fairly large in *Leechbook III* and in *Lacnunga*, it is relatively small in Bald's *Leechbook*, indicating that a more sophisticated compiler or practitioner was less likely to resort to magical practices in medicine and to rely more on remedies which were rationally conceived. But to understand all ancient and medieval medicine one must try to understand the part played in it by magical and superstitious practices. So we will next examine the magical element of Anglo-Saxon medicine in order to see its role in their treatment of disease.

[53] Bonser, *Medical Background*, p. 35.   [54] *Ibid.*, p. 8.

13

Magical medicine

Like that of all ancient and medieval societies, Anglo-Saxon medicine had a large component of magic, and in the recent past the magical elements have received more attention than the rational ones. Although magic played a smaller part in it than is implied by many commentators, it is an integral and interesting part and deserves a sympathetic assessment. I mentioned in previous chapters that magical remedies were most commonly prescribed for conditions which were intractable to rational treatments; this implies that they were resorted to for conditions where rational remedies had proved ineffective.

Dysentery, for example, was a difficult condition to treat successfully and many remedies for it are magical in whole or in part; here is a typical one combining rational and magical features, which we may keep in mind in the discussion which follows:

For dysentery: a bramble of which both ends are in the ground; take the newer root, dig up, cut off nine shavings into the left hand and sing three times *Miserere mei, Deus*, and nine times *Pater Noster*, then take mugwort and everlasting; boil the three in milk until they are done; then sip after a night's fast a good dishful a while before he eats other food; let him rest quietly and wrap him up warm. If more is needed, do the same again, then if you still need it, do it a third time; you will not need to more often.[1]

The magical components are the tip-rooted shoot and the reciting of the *Miserere* and *Pater Noster*; the rest is a rational herbal treatment for diarrhoea or dysentery. Of the bramble, Mrs Grieve wrote:

[1] *Leechdoms*, ed. Cockayne II, 290–2: 'Wiþ utwærce: brembel þe sien begen endas on eorþan, genim þone neowran wyrttruman, delf up, þwit nigon sponas on þa winstran hand 7 sing þriwa miserere mei deus 7 nigon siþum pater noster, genim þonne mucgwyrt 7 efelastan, wyl þas þreo on meolcum oþ þæt hy readian, supe þonne on neahtnestig gode

130

The bark of the root and the leaves contain much tannin, and have long been esteemed as a capital astringent and tonic, proving a valuable remedy for dysentery and diarrhoea, etc. . . . The root bark, used medicinally, should be peeled off the root . . . One ounce, boiled in 1½ pint water or milk down to a pint, makes a good decoction. Half a teacupful should be taken every hour or two for diarrhoea.[2]

Modern herbals do not recommend mugwort for loose bowels. If *efelasten* is the same plant as life everlasting or catsfoot (*Antennaria* spp.) then it too was useful; it is 'said to be efficacious . . . for looseness of bowels'.[3] On strictly rational grounds, the potion should have done some good but, dysentery being a difficult ailment to treat, resort was had to irrational elements as well.

Although it is not easy to give a strict definition of magic, we will find it helpful in this discussion to use a statement by Nöth:

The magician's semiotic fallacy is based on his neglecting the principle of independence between the sign and the 'thing' referred to. The sign and the 'thing' referred to are not considered as independent entities but as something forming an undifferentiated unity. In magic, this confusion of the dimensions of 'object' and 'sign' is accompanied by an additional assumption; it is expected that a manipulation of the sign (more exactly a signifier) causes a simultaneous transformation of the 'thing'.[4]

Nöth has also pointed out that in Anglo-Saxon medical records there are three types of remedies: (1) those containing a magic act and a magic formula; (2) those containing a magic act but no magic formula; and (3) those having no magic features.[5] In this chapter we will deal with types (1) and (2), although it may at times be difficult to distinguish between a remedy of type (2) and type (3), our decision depending to a great extent on whether we believe that a remedy was used because of its supposedly magical powers or because it was conceived by its users as wholly rational, the application of its ingredients having been found effective against specific ailments. Distinction of types may also be influenced by the fact that a magical remedy may be of more help to the patient than a rational one. We must guard against finding magical connotations in remedies which to their users were not thought to be magical.

blede fulle hwile he oþerne mete þicge; reste hine softe 7 wreo hine wearme. Gif ma þearf sie do eft swa, gif þu þonne git þurfe do þriddan siþe; ne þearft þu oftor.'
2 Grieve, *A Modern Herbal*, pp. 109–10.   3 *Ibid.*, p. 175.
4 Nöth, 'Semiotics', pp. 59–83, at p. 66.
5 *Ibid.*, p. 62.

It will be convenient to examine magical remedies according to their various forms, and we can begin most easily with a relatively small group, the amulets. Because 'amulet' may have various meanings, I shall use it here to mean simply something *worn or carried about the body or kept in one's dwelling for therapeutic or healing purposes*, but not as a medicine to be applied to the body as a poultice or plaster or to be taken internally. As an example of an amulet defined in this way, here is a remedy from *Leechbook III*: 'For pain in the jaw: take the spindle with which a woman spins, bind around his neck with a woollen thread and rinse the inside with hot goat's milk; he will soon be well.'[6] The spindle tied to the neck is an amulet; the hot goat's milk is a rational medicine, recommended by Pliny and Marcellus as a gargle for sore throat and toothache. On the other hand, the next remedy in the same chapter is what appears to be an amulet with no rational component: 'For sore throat dig up plantain before sunrise, tie on his neck.'[7]

In ch. 6 we quoted an amuletic remedy recommended in *Leechbook III*, namely, the eyes of a live crab tied around the neck of someone who has swollen eyes. Another amulet from the same work is for temptations of the devil: 'For temptation of the devil, there is a herb called *rud molin* which grows by running water; if you have it on you and under your pillow and over the door of your house the devil cannot harm you indoors or out.'[8] Cockayne identified *rud molin* as water pepper (*Polygonum hydropiper*), on the assumption that the name was an error for *rudniolin* ('red stalk'), an Old Norse plant name quite suitable for the water plant described in the remedy, and because water pepper has the dialectal name 'redshanks' in English. He is probably correct, although the related amphibious bistort (*P. amphibium*) fits the description just as well. If Cockayne was right in his identification, then the compiler (or scribe) of the *Leechbook* or some predecessor was not familiar with the name and misspelled it. This implies that this amulet was not of native English origin, but was borrowed from the Scandinavians.

---

[6] *Leechdoms*, ed. Cockayne II, 310–12: 'Við ceocadle nim þone hweorfan þe wif mid spinnað, bind on his sweoran mid wyllenan þræde 7 swile innan mid hate gate meolce; him biþ sel.'

[7] *Ibid.*, p. 312: 'Wiþ ceol wærce adelf ær sunnan upgange wegbrædan, bind on his sweoran.'

[8] *Ibid.*, p. 342: 'Wiþ feondes costunge rud molin hatte wyrt weaxeþ be yrnendum wætre; gif þu þa on þe hafast 7 under þinum heafodbolstre 7 ofer þines huses durum ne mæg þe deofol sceþþan inne ne ute.'

The number of amuletic remedies in Anglo-Saxon records is not large and most of them are in *Leechbook III*. The following is an interesting one from Bald's *Leechbook*: 'For much travelling over land, lest he tire let him take mugwort in his hand or in his shoe lest he become weary; and when he will take it before sunrise let him say these words first: "I take thee artemisia lest I be tired on the road." Make the sign of the cross on it when you pull it up.'[9] In this recipe, not only is the mugwort used as an amulet; magical formulas are also attached to the gathering of it. It is found in much simpler form in Pliny: 'A traveller who has mugwort and sage tied on him is said not to feel fatigue.'[10] It is not clear whether Pliny recommended either mugwort *or* sage or whether his recipe required both. It is in the *Herbarium* also in a simple form: 'If anyone making a journey carries mugwort with him in his hand he will not feel the weariness of the journey.'[11] As late as the nineteenth century Fernie wrote: 'If placed in the shoes, it will prevent weariness.'[12]

There were also Christian amulets; here is one from Bald's *Leechbook* for *lencten adl* ('spring fever', or endemic tertian malaria): 'Again a divine prayer: In nomine domini summi sit benedictum. ⋈MMRMþ . N7 . þTX⋈MRFpN7 . þTX. Again one shall in silence write this and put the words in silence on the left breast, and let him not go in (doors) with that writing nor carry it in (doors), and also put this on in silence: HΛMMΛNy°EL . BPONice . NOy°epTΛy°EpΓ.'[13] The runic words ⋈MMRMþ . N7 . þTX⋈MRFpN7 . þTX. have been interpreted by Cockayne as 'DEEREþ HAND þIN DEREþ HAND þIN' by reading the 'T' as an 'I'; this he translated as 'thine hand vexeth, thine hand vexeth'. The final

---

9 *Ibid.*, p. 154: 'Wiþ miclum gonge ofer land, þy læs he teorige: mucgwyrt nime him on hand oþþe do on his sco þy læs he meþige: 7 þonne he niman wille ær sunnan upgange cweþe þas word ærest: "Tollam te artemesia ne lassus sum in uia"; gesena hie þonne þu up teo.'

10 Pliny, *HN* XXVI.150: 'Artemisiam et elelisphacum alligatas qui habeat viator negatur lassitudinem sentire.'

11 *Herbarium*, ed. de Vriend, pp. 55–7: 'Herba artemisia monoclonos, si quis iter faciens eam secum in manu portaverit non sentiet itineris laborem.'

12 Fernie, *Old Fashioned Herbal Remedies*, p. 325.

13 *Leechdoms*, ed. Cockayne II, 140: 'Eft godcunde gebed. In nomine domini summi sit benedictum. ⋈MMRMþ . N7 . þTX⋈MRFpN7 . þTX. Eft sceal mon swigende þis writan 7 don þas word swigende on þa winstran breost 7 ne ga he in on þæt gewrit ne in on ber, 7 eac swigende þis on don: HΛMMΛNy°EL . BPONice . NOy°epTΛy°EpΓ.' (In Cockayne's transcript the words 'domini summi' are omitted and the last 'þ' is written 'R'.)

words seem to be an attempt to write *Emmanuel* and *Veronica* and a third undecipherable word or phrase all in Greek letters. Here we find basically Christian elements combined with pagan symbols (the runic letters). Emmanuel was a name of great potency against spirits in the Middle Ages; Veronica was the compassionate woman who wiped Christ's face on the way to Calvary and found his image on her cloth afterwards; it is almost as if the magician was hedging his bets by invoking both heathen and Christian aids.

In *Lacnunga* there are a couple of remedies containing charms to be written down and attached to the sufferer. In the remedy *Wið dweorg*, the charm was to be hung about the patient's neck by a virgin (this charm is discussed in detail below, p. 151). Another for diarrhoea is worth quoting in full: 'For diarrhoea: this epistle the angel brought to Rome, when they were greatly afflicted with diarrhoea; write this on a piece of vellum as long as may surround the head outside and hang it on the neck of the person who has need of it. He will soon be well: "Ranmigan . . . Alleluia."'[14] The charm words are unintelligible although among them may be recognized Latin words and phrases, Greek words and what may be a few in Hebrew. Doubtless their unintelligibility contributed to their magical efficacy.

When is an amulet not an amulet? It is sometimes very difficult to be sure whether a remedy is amuletic or rational in intent. Consider this one, also from *Lacnunga*: 'For a woman struck suddenly dumb: take pennyroyal and grind to powder and wrap up in wool; put under the woman; she will soon be well.'[15] At first glance, this looks very much like a typical amulet, but further consideration leads to the impression that it is a purely rational remedy. Why should a woman be struck suddenly dumb? Cassius Felix wrote: 'Suffocation of the womb is followed by sudden illness, loss of voice

[14] Grattan and Singer, *Anglo-Saxon Magic*, p. 188: 'Wið utsihte: þysne pistol se ængel brohte to rome, þa hy wæran mid utsihte micclum geswæncte: writ þis on swa langum bocfelle þæt hit mæge befon utan þæt heafod 7 hoh on þæs mannes sweoran þe him þearf sy; him bið sona sel: "Ranmigan adonai. eltheos. mur. O ineffabile. Omiginan. midanmian. misane. dimas. mode. mida. memagartem. Orta min. sigmone. beronice. irritas. uenas quasi dulaþ. feruor. fruxantis. sanguinis. siccatur. fla fracta. frigula. mirgui. etsihdon. segulta. frautantur. in arno. midoninis. abar uetho. sydone multo. saccula pp pppp sother sother. miserere mei deus deus mini deus mi. Amen Alleluia Alleluia."'

[15] *Ibid.*, p. 180: 'Wið ðon ðe wif færunga adumbige: genim pollegian 7 gnid to duste 7 in wulle bewind; alege under þæt wif; hyre bið sona sel.'

so that they are dumb.'[16] Pennyroyal is an emmenagogue; Dioscorides recommended it in a sitz-bath (i.e., as a topical application, not as a potion) for 'inflations and hardnesses and aversions' of the womb.[17] In our recipe it seems to be a pessary of pennyroyal in wool (i.e., put under the woman) to treat suppression of menses; if so, it is not an amulet.

Examples enough have been given to show that amulets played no small part in Anglo-Saxon medicine. There are also many amuletic remedies in the *Herbarium*; but the *Herbarium* is not an originally English compilation and it is impossible to decide which of its remedies actually entered the English repertory of treatments except where they are found in other Old English contexts as well.

As we have just seen, it is not always easy to determine whether a remedy is magic or not when it is not accompanied by a magic formula (Nöth's type (2)). Is the following one, already quoted, magical or rational? 'Against a woman's mad behaviour: eat a radish before breakfast and that day the madness cannot bother you.'[18] Was the radish supposed to protect one from the *gemædla* or was it supposed to give one a mental equanimity immune to distraction? The first suggestion would be a magic act, the second not necessarily so. But there are others where the magical act is clear. The first remedy of *Leechbook III*, already quoted, for headache required that the medicine be tied to the head with a *red* fillet; the colour requirement can only be magical. Similarly, in the following example, it must be for a magical reason that the whip was made of porpoise skin: 'In case one is moonsick, take porpoise skin, make into a whip, beat the man with it, he will soon be well.'[19] To this remedy someone (in a hand other than that of the scribe) added the word 'amen'.

Here is another remedy which, on the face of it, seems to be magical: 'For headache, hound's head, burn to ashes and shave the head, lay on.'[20] Nöth quoted it as an example of his type (2), a magical act without magical

---

[16] *Cassii Felicis De Medicina* , ed. Rose, p. 187: 'Praefocationem matricis sequitur subitus casus, vocis amputatio ut obmutescant.'

[17] *Dioscuridis de Materia Medica*, ed. Wellmann III, 41: εἰς ἐνκάθισμα πρὸς ἐμπνευματώσεις καὶ σκληρίας καὶ ἀποστροφὰς ὑστέρα ('It is good in a vapour bath for inflations and hardnesses and aversions of the womb.').

[18] *Leechdoms*, ed. Cockayne II, 342: 'Wiþ wif gemædlan geberge on neahtnestig rædices moran; þy dæge ne mæg þe se gemædla sceþþan.'

[19] *Ibid.*, p. 334: 'Wiþ þon þe mon sie monaþ seoc nim mereswines fel, wyrc to swipan. swing mid þone man, sona biδ sel.'

[20] *Ibid.*, p. 20: 'Wiδ heafodece hundes heafod gebærn to ahsan 7 sniδ þæt heafod, lege on.'

formula;[21] and Storms commented: 'In pronouncing a comparison the magician supposes the two elements to be similar in hopes to make them similar. The idea that two objects are connected with each other may be based on similarity in sound, meaning, form, colour and so on.'[22] Nöth wrote: 'The text reports a magic act since the effectiveness of the remedy is evidently believed to rely on the relationship of similarity between the therapeutic act on the one hand and the process of recovery on the other: just as the dog's head burns to ashes, the headache is believed to vanish.'[23] The arguments of both commentators depend on the interpretation of the words *hundes heafod* and both have takan them to mean the head of a dog. But there is another *hundes heafod* in medieval medicine, the snapdragon, *Antirrhinum orontium*, prescribed in the *Herbarium* for excessive watering of the eyes[24] and which is still prescribed in herbal medicine to treat ulcers, skin eruptions and haemorrhoids. It is now impossible to decide between plant and animal origin for the ashes of 'hound's head', so that we cannot know whether the remedy was magical or rational to its medieval users.

For other remedies the claim for magical intent cannot be maintained. Storms[25] attributed the magical concept of similarity to this one: 'For distress of the stomach . . . rub pennyroyal in vinegar and water, give to drink, soon the distress goes away.'[26] Storms translated *magan wærce* by 'heartburn' and commented: 'There is the notion of similarity: the sharp sour taste of vinegar is employed against the sharp sour taste produced by heartburn.' But the Old English recipe is a direct descendant of one given by Marcellus for what he called *nausea stomachi* ('nausea of the stomach'),[27] and followed one given by Dioscorides 'for nausea and gnawings of the stomach'.[28] Gerard wrote: 'Pennie Royal . . . taken with water and vinegar asswageth the inordinate desire to vomite, & the pains of the stomach.'[29] It is very doubtful that the *magan wærce* of the Old English recipe was heartburn rather than digestive distress in the stomach. Now pennyroyal has had a long and well-deserved reputation as a carminative and is still used to relieve a distressed stomach; like the more commonly

[21] Nöth, 'Semiotics', pp. 63–4.   [22] Storms, *Anglo-Saxon Magic*, p. 56.

[23] Nöth, 'Semiotics', p. 64.

[24] *Herbarium*, ed. de Vriend, p. 127.   [25] Storms, *Anglo-Saxon Magic*, p. 70.

[26] *Leechdoms*, ed. Cockayne II, 356: 'Wiþ magan wærce . . . gnid on eced 7 on wæter polleian, sele drincan. sona þæt sar toglit.'

[27] *Marcelli De Medicamentis*, ed. Niedermann, p. 334.

[28] *Dioscuridis de Materia Medica*, ed. Wellmann II, 41: ναυσίας τε καὶ δηγμούς στομάχου.

[29] Gerard, *The Herball*, p. 672.

used mint, it is prepared in dilute vinegar. So it is most unlikely that the remedy was magical to its users.

I have already mentioned that magical remedies were resorted to for conditions treated with difficulty by rational means. This is shown very well by a chapter in Bald's *Leechbook* on haemorrhage from the nose:

(1) If blood run from one's nose too much: take green betony and rue, pound in vinegar, twist together the same as a sloe, thrust into the nose. (2) Blood stancher: bishop's wort the lower part, eat or drink in milk. (3) Blood stancher, again: take hedge clivers, bind on the neck. (4) Blood stancher, again: springwort, put in the ear . . . (5) Blood stancher again: a whole ear of barley, thrust into the ear so that he is not aware of it. (6) Blood stancher, again: Some write this: '+ ægryn . . . aeR. leNo.'; either for horse or for man a blood stancher.[30]

Of these remedies, only the first two appear to be rational, whether effective or not. Both betony and rue are recommended in the *Herbarium* for nosebleed. It is difficult to see how putting things in the ear or around the neck would stop bleeding from the nose. Remedy no. 5 may be an exception; although it appears that the ear of barley thrust into the ear of the person is an example of contiguity of names conferring a magical efficacy, it is also just possible that the sudden startle caused by the thrusting of a barley ear secretly into a patient's ear would bring about the 'fight or flight' reaction of adrenalin release with consequent constriction of peripheral blood vessels, permitting more effective clotting to take place. Remedy no. 6 is tantalizing for the questions it raises; on what was the writing done, how was it used? There is about it an air of scepticism, as if the compiler doubted its usefulness: 'Sume þis writað', but not everyone thinks it worthwhile. This chapter well illustrates the ambivalent approach to magical remedies which we find in Bald's *Leechbook*.

The magical component of a remedy may reside in the use of ingredients which have been consecrated to a religious use: 'For one who is devil-sick:

---

[30] *Leechdoms*, ed. Cockayne II, 54: '(1) Gif men yrne blod of nebbe to swiðe genim grene betonican 7 rudan, gecnuwa on eced, gwring tosomne swilce sie an slah, sting on þa nosu. (2) Blod seten: bisceop wyrt nioþowearde, ete oððe on meolce drince. (3) Blod seten eft: genim hegeclifan, gebinde on sweoran. (4) Blod seten eft: springwyrt, do on eare. (5) Blod seten eft: gehal beren ear bestinge on eare swa he nyte. (6) Sume þis writað: + ægryn. thon. struth. fola argrenn. tart. struth. on. tria. enn. piath. hathu. morfana. on hæl + ara. carn. leou. groth. weorn. †††. ffil. crondi. p. ⋈. mro. cron. ærcrio. ermio. aeR. leNo.; ge horse ge men blod seten.'

put in holy-water and in ale bishopwort, hindheal, agrimony, alexanders, cockle, give him to drink.'[31] Again: 'If any harmful temptation come on one, either an elf or a night-goer, anoint his face with this salve and put on his eyes and where his body is sore and cense him and sign him [with the cross] frequently; his condition will soon be better.'[32]

Although remedies such as these are magical to our way of thinking, we should ask ourselves if they were thought to be so by their medieval users. Even today a practising Christian will see nothing magical or superstitious in prayers for rain as part of a church service, while looking on an Indian rain dance as a magical performance. To many of us, the use of holy water, of consecrated wine and salt and oil of extreme unction is a magical, or at least a superstitious, practice. The consecration of these substances had dedicated them to a special use in Christian ceremonies and sacraments, and they could all easily be believed to have undergone a substantial transformation by such dedication, just as the bread and wine of the eucharist became the flesh and blood of Christ. So, after their consecration, they must have been substantially different from what they had been before, no longer being simply bread, wine, salt and oil, and in their new guises might be expected to have medicinal properties different from their original ones. If this view of medieval belief in the effects of consecration of substances is acceptable, then the amount of truly magical behaviour (from the point of view of the medieval practitioner) was much less than it appears to us.

The following remedy shows the extent to which ritualistic healing could go:

For elfsickness, take bishopswort, fennel, lupin, alfthone the lower part and lichen from a hallowed crucifix and frankincense, put a handful of each, tie up all the herbs in a cloth, dip in consecrated font-water three times, let sing over them three masses: one, *Omnibus sanctis*, another, *Contra tribulationem*, the third, *Pro infirmis*; then put coals in a brazier and lay the herbs on them, then cense the man with the herbs before tierce and at night and sing the *Litany* and *Creed* and *Pater Noster* and write a Christ's cross for him on every limb, and take a little handful of herbs of

[31] *Leechdoms*, ed. Cockayne II, 354: 'Viþ deofol seoce: do on halig wæter 7 on eala bisceopwyrte, hindhioloþan, agrimonian, alexandrian, gyþrifan, sele him drincan.'
[32] *Ibid.*, p. 344: 'Gif men hwilc yfel costung weorþe, oþþe ælf oþþe nihtgengan, smire his andwlitan mid þisse sealfe 7 on his eagan do 7 þær him se lichoman sar sie 7 recelsa hine 7 sena gelome his þing biþ sona selre.'

these same kinds similarly consecrated and boil in milk, drip holy water on them three times and let sup before his meal; he will soon be well.[33]

Even more elaborate is this one:

If he has the *elfsogoþa* [Cockayne translated 'elf hiccup'; Geldner suggested 'elf-sucked', i.e., 'anaemic'], his eyes are yellow where they should be red. If you wish to treat the man, consider his behaviour and observe which sex he is: if it is a male and he looks up when you first examine him and his face is dark yellow, that man you might cure completely if he has not been too long in it; if it is a woman and she looks down when you first examine her and her face is dusky red, you may treat her also. If it is longer by a day than twelve months and the appearance be like this, then you can improve it for a while, and yet cannot cure completely. Write this writing: *Scriptum est rex regum et dominus dominantium. byrnice. beronice. luslure. iehe. aius. aius. aius. Sanctus. Sanctus. Sanctus. dominus deus Sabaoth. amen. aleluiah.* Sing this over the drink and the writing: *Deus omnipotens pater domini nostri ihesu christi. per inpositionem huius scriptura expelle a famulo tuo N. omnem impetum castalidum, de capite, de capillis, de cerebro, de fronte, de lingua, de sublingua, de guttore, de faucibus, de dentibus, de oculis, de naribus, de auribus, de manibus, de collo, de brachiis, de corde, de anima, de genibus, de coxis, de pedibus, de compaginibus omnium membrorum intus et foris. amen.* Then make a drink: font water, rue, sage, cassock, dracontia, smooth plantain the lower part, feverfew, dill blossoms, three cloves of garlic, fennel, wormwood, lovage, lupin, all of equal amounts; write three time a cross with oil of extreme unction and say: *Pax tibi.* Then take the writing, with it write a cross over the drink and sing this over it: *Deus omnipotens pater domini nostri ihesu Christi per inpositionem huius scriptura et per gustum huius expelle diabolum a famulo tuo N.*; and the *Credo* and *Pater Noster*. Wet the writing in the drink, and write a cross with it on each limb and say: *Signum crucis Christi conservate in vitam eternam amen.* If you do not wish to, bid the patient himself or one who is most closely related to him, and let him cross him as best as he can. This treatment is good for every temptation of the devil.[34]

---

[33] *Ibid.*, pp. 344–6: 'Wið ælfadle nim bisceopwyrt, finul, elehtre, ælfþonan nioþowearde 7 gehalgodes cristes mæles ragu 7 stor, do ælcre handfulle, bebind ealle þa wyrta on claþe, bedyp on fontwætre gehalgodum þriwa, læt singan ofer .III. mæssan: ane omnibus Sanctis, oþre contra tribulationem, þriddan pro infirmis; do þonne gleda an gledfæt 7 lege þa wyrta on, gerec þone man mid þam wyrtum ær undern 7 on niht 7 sing letania 7 credan 7 pater noster 7 writ him cristes mæl on ælcum lime, 7 nim lytle handfulle þæs ilcan cynnes wyrta gelice gehalgode 7 wyl on meolce, dryp þriwa gehalgodes wætres on 7 supe ær his mete; him biþ sona sel.'

[34] *Ibid.*, pp. 348–50; see Appendix 2 (below, p. 191).

There is more than one interesting feature to this elaborate remedy. It is one of the few in the Old English repertory to have a prognosis of illness based on the appearance of the patient. It combines (as do other magical remedies) quite rational medicines with elaborate magical rituals. It contains a lorica-like prayer, enumerating in order all parts of the body to be protected from the assaults of elves, which in the Latin invocation are called *castalides*, that is, *dunælfen* ('mountain-elves'). The suggestion at the end that the operator may not wish to carry out the whole of the procedure is puzzling; is the operator a cleric who may think it improper to do what the procedure requires, or is there an element of danger in it which he wishes to avoid? And why should it be done instead only by the patient or a near relative? There are questions for which we should like to have answers, but none are forthcoming.

Among the Old English magical remedies several metrical charms are not only of great interest but of literary value also. Many are in a more or less corrupt state and are also usually difficult or even impossible of certain interpretation. They have consequently been edited and commented on in numerous attempts to elucidate them; in the following notes I shall try to express the most useful of these attempts.

A half dozen of them are in the *Lacnunga*, and of these the most striking is that given under the title *Wið færstice*. It opens with directions in prose giving the ingredients and method of preparation of a medicine, followed by the metrical charm proper and closes with final directions in prose for administration of the medicine:[35]

For a sudden stitch: Feverfew and the red nettle that grows in through the corn and plantain, boil in butter.

Loud were they, yea loud, when they rode over the hill [grave mound],
were of one mind [fierce] when they rode over the land.
Shield thou now thyself, that thou mayest survive this attack [affliction].   5
Out, little spear, if thou be herein.
[I] stood under linden, under a light shield,
where the mighty women made ready their powers,
and spears yelling they sent.
I will send another back to them, a flying arrow in opposition to them.   10
Out, little spear, if it be herein.
A smith sat, forged a knife;
small the iron, mighty the wound.

[35] Grattan and Singer, *Anglo-Saxon Magic*, pp. 172–6; see Appendix 2 (below, pp. 191–2).

Out, little spear, if it be herein.   15
Six smiths sat, wrought battle-spears.
Out, spear, not in, spear.
If herein be a bit of iron, work of witches, it shall melt.
If thou wert shot in skin, or wert shot in flesh,   20
or wert shot in blood, or wert shot in limb,
never would thy life be smitten.
If it were shot of gods, or if it were shot of elves,
or if it were shot of witches, now I shall help thee.
This be to thee as a remedy for shot of gods,   25
this be to thee as a remedy for shot of elves,
this be to thee as a remedy for shot of witches; I will help thee.
Fled there on the mountain top.
Be thou healthy; may the Lord help thee.

Then take the knife, apply the liquid.

An analysis of this charm may prove useful, because the principles of charm medicine which emerge here can be applied to Anglo-Saxon medical charms in general. It appears to be purely pagan; only in the last line the words 'may the Lord help thee' may be a reference to the Christian God. This being so, it can give us information about pre-Christian medical beliefs and practices of the Anglo-Saxons. But first some comment on the received text is necessary.

The word *færstice* is found only in this charm. Cockayne, Grendon and Grattan and Singer translated it literally as 'sudden stitch'; Grendon added in a note, 'intended to cure a sudden twinge or stitch, possibly rheumatism, supposedly due to shots sent by witches, elves, and other spirits flying through the air';[36] Grattan and Singer gave it the supplementary title *Pagan Lay for Elfshot*,[37] which is clearly incorrect, as elves are only one of three agents held responsible for the ailment; Storms gave 'rheumatism'.[38] Considering how little information we have, Storms's gloss seems to me to be too precise. It is more probable that *færstice* meant any sudden pain anywhere in the body, such as a muscular cramp, a joint pain (which might be rheumatism), a 'stitch in the side' from overexertion, or even an angina pain or lumbago. It may be significant that *Hexenschuss* (literally, 'witch-shot') is the German word for 'lumbago', a rheumatic pain

---

[36] Grendon, 'Anglo-Saxon Charms', pp. 105–237, at 165 and 214.

[37] Grattan and Singer, *Anglo-Saxon Magic*, p. 175.

[38] Storms, *Anglo-Saxon Magic*, pp. 158–63; see esp. pp. 160–1.

(often of sudden onset) in the lumbar region. There is good evidence that many ailments which appear suddenly were once thought to be caused by elves or witches shooting arrows at the sufferer. An illustration in the Eadwine Psalter shows a man who is being attacked by small winged creatures and whose skin is covered with spots, some of them pierced by arrows (Cambridge, Trinity College R. 17. 1 (987), 66r). This is most probably an example of *elfshot*. In another set of magical remedies we will see that *ælfadl* ('elf-sickness') is most probably chicken-pox, and in others that it is some other eruption on the skin. In the present charm, the attack of elves (or other malignant spirits) results in sudden pains in muscles or joints.

This belief in elfshots seems to have been widespread; Alexander Carmichael found a charm in the Scottish Highlands which was for *galar toll*, a pain which struck 'before and behind the shoulder' and for which a remedy was to rub the painful places *an t-saighead shith a chur 'na tosd* ('to still the fairy arrows').[39] But it is not clear that Anglo-Saxon physicians by the time of Bald and later still believed that some ailments were caused by attacks of elves; *Hexenschuss* ('witch-shot') raises no vision of witches in the minds of Germans today when they use it to refer to lumbago.

The prose preface gives a recipe for a salve to treat *færstice*. The ingredients are feverfew, red nettle, plantain and butter. *Feferfuige* is not easy to identify. Based on the Old English translation of the *Herbarium*, it has been equated with *Centaurium umbellatum*, where it is described as 'Curmelle, feferfuge, centauria minor'.[40] This is the only instance in Old English where *feferfuge* (*feferfuige*) is compared with a Latin plant name. But we should bear in mind that in *Lacnunga* lxxxvib,[41] *curmel* and *feferfugean* are both prescribed in the same recipe, and also that the Old English *Herbarium* does not always correctly identify the plants of its Latin original. So it is possible that *feferfuige* may have been the plant now called 'feverfew' (*Chrysanthemum parthenium*). Whichever it may have been is not of great importance, as both species have been prescribed by herbalists for the relief of rheumatic and other pains.

I have translated *seo reade netele ðe þurh ærn inwyx* by 'the red nettle that grows in through the corn'. Most editors and commentators have given 'the red nettle which grows through the house' (Grendon), 'the red nettle which grows through [the wall of] a house' (Storms), 'the red nettle that groweth through into a house' (Grattan and Singer). If the plant is to be identified as

---

[39] *Carmina*, ed. Carmichael IV, 306–7.   [40] *Herbarium*, ed. de Vriend, p. 82.
[41] Grattan and Singer, *Anglo-Saxon Magic*, p. 158.

a species of *Urtica* (family Urticaceae), Cockayne's is the best rendering, as true nettles, especially *Urtica urens*, often grow near buildings, especially on middens where there is litter and rubble. The problem with this identification is that true nettles are not red. As we saw in ch. 11, the plant usually called *red nettle* or *red dead-nettle* is *Lamium purpureum* (family Labiatae), whose leaves bear a superficial resemblance to those of the true nettles, but lack their stinging hairs (hence *dead*), has reddish colour in its leaves, particularly the smaller upper ones and bears pinkish–purple flowers. True nettles do not seem to have been prescribed for muscular aches and pains, whereas the dead-nettles 'give ease in gout, sciatica and other pains in the joints and muscles', when applied as a salve in lard, etc., according to a modern herbal.[42]

Lamium purpureum, while very common in cultivated ground and waste places, does not tend to grow around buildings. It has been suggested that *ærn* in this recipe does not mean 'house', but is a form of *earnð, ærnð,* meaning 'corn', 'crop of corn', so that the meaning may be 'the red nettle which grows in through the corn'.[43] This interpretation is particularly interesting in view of a remark by Mrs Grieve:

> The plant [red dead-nettle] varies greatly in appearance, according to the situation in which it grows. On the open ground, it is somewhat spreading in habit rarely more than 6 inches in height, whilst specimens growing in the midst of crowded vegetation are often drawn up to a considerable height, their leaves being of a dull green throughout, whereas those of the smaller specimens grown in the open are ordinarily more or less warm and rich in colour. At first glance the variation in the appearance of specimens grown under these different circumstances would leave the casual observer to suppose them to belong to different species.[44]

That is, specimens growing in crowded places would look more like true nettles than those growing on open ground. It is possible that this had been noticed by the Anglo-Saxons and that the reference to habitat in the recipe was intended to designate the type of *red nettle* to be used.

Of the other plants, *wegbræde* is a plantain, most likely the common plantain, (*Plantago maior*). Plantain was an ingredient of a multitude of remedies; in the *Herbarium* it was recommended for gout, for pain or swelling of sinews, for sore feet, etc.[45] All three herbs have been

---

[42] Grieve, *A Modern Herbal*, pp. 578–9 and 582.

[43] F. P. Magoun, Jr, 'Zu den ae. Zaubersprüchen', *Archiv* 171 (1937), 17–35.

[44] Grieve, *A Modern Herbal*, p. 581.   [45] *Herbarium*, ed. de Vriend, p. 41.

recommended for muscular and joint pains, hence useful against 'sudden stitch', when applied as a salve to the aching parts.

The function of the charm was to exorcise an attack by malignant creatures, to cause their arrows to leave the patient. The exorcist gave confidence to the patient by describing the onset of a host riding over a grave-mound, by asserting that he had a stronger medicine with which to oppose the host, and by describing the forging of a knife which will act against the weapons of the attackers. He next enumerated the parts of the body subject to attack and the identities of possible attackers so that all eventualities were covered. Then, taking the herbs one by one, he declared each a remedy for attack by one malignant being or another before putting it into the boiling butter. Finally, he declared that the attacker had fled to the mountain top and that with the Lord's help the pain would be relieved. Then, using the knife, he applied the salve.

Even without the charm, the hot salve should have had some effect on the pain of a sudden stitch, and the rigmarole of the charm gave added assurance to the patient that the remedy would work.

The second charm to be considered is the one most editors have named *The Nine Herbs Charm*.[46] Its text is very corrupt, there being omissions and transpositions of existing parts, but the general meaning is clear and we can learn something more about early Anglo-Saxon medical beliefs by examining it. In the manuscript the charm is preceded by one remedy for *fig* ('haemorrhoids') and followed by two more for the same ailment.

Because of the corrupt condition of the charm in the manuscript, any translation must be tentative; the following one keeps to the transmitted text as closely as possible:

> Keep in mind mugwort, what you revealed,
> What you established at Regenmelde.
> You are called Una, oldest of herbs,
> You have power against three and against thirty,
> You have power against poison and against infection,   5
> You have power against the loathsome one who roams through the land.
> +   And you, plantain, mother of herbs,
> Open from the east, mighty within,
> Over you carts have run, over you queens have ridden,

---

[46] Grattan and Singer, *Anglo-Saxon Magic*, pp. 150–6; see Appendix 2 (below, pp. 192–4). Anyone who doubts the psychological value to the patient of this and the preceding charm, *Wiŏ færstice*, should try chanting them aloud; they have a marvellously incantatory effect.

Over you brides have cried out, over you bulls have snorted.   10
All have you then withstood and do confound;
So may you withstand poison and infection
And the loathsome thing that roams through the land.
   This herb is called *stune*, it has grown on stone;
She stands against poison, she dashes against suffering,   15
She is called stiff, she dashes against poison,
She expels malignant things, casts out poison.
+   This is the herb which fought with the serpent,
It has power against poison, it has power against infection,
It has power against the loathsome thing that roams through the land.   20
Do you now put to flight, attorlothe, the lesser the greater,
The greater the lesser, until he has a remedy from both.
   Keep in mind, chamomile, what you revealed,
What you brought to pass at Alorford,
That never for infection was life surrendered   25
Since one had mayweed made ready for him for food.
   This the herb which is called *wergulu*,
The seal sent it over the sea's ridge
As a cure for the injury of another poison.
   These nine goads against nine poisons.   30
+   A serpent came crawling, it wounded no one.
Then Woden took nine glorious twigs,
Struck then that adder so that she flew apart into nine pieces.
There apple and poison made an end
That she never should dwell in a house.   35
+   Chervil and fennel, very mighty two,
These herbs the wise Lord created,
Holy in heaven where he hung,
Ordained and sent into the seven worlds,
For poor and for rich, a cure for all.   40
   She stands against pain, she assaults poison,
She has power against three and against thirty,
Against the hand of fiend and against the hand against mighty tricks
Against enchantment by evil things.
+   Now the nine herbs have power against nine fled from glory,   45
Against nine poisons and against nine infections,
Against the red poison, against the foul poison,
Against the white poison, against the purple poison,
Against the yellow poison, against the green poison,
Against the lurid poison, against the purple poison,   50

145

Against the brown poison, against the blue poison,
Against serpent blister, against water blister,
Against thorn blister, against this[tle] blister,
Against ice blister, against poison blister.
If any poison come flying from the east,   55
Or any come from the north,
Or any from the west over the human race,
+ Christ stood over old oppressive ones.
    I alone know the running waters
And the nine adders they restrain.   60
Now must all weeds spring up as herbs,
Seas slip away, all salt water,
When I blow this poison from you.

Mugwort, plantain which is open from the east, lamb's cress, attorlothe, chamomile, nettle, crab apple, chervil and fennel, old soap. Work the plants to powder, mix with the soap and with the pulped apple. Make a paste of water and of ashes, take the fennel, boil in the paste and foment with the ?mixture? when the salve is applied, both before and after. Sing the charm on each of the herbs, three times before he works them up and on the apple also, and let someone sing in the mouth and in both ears and on the wound the same charm before the salve is applied.

Grattan and Singer gave the charm the title *Pagan Lay of the Nine Herbs*; and attempts at interpretation have almost invariably assumed that it was originally pagan and minimally Christianized by the introduction of Christ's name in line 58 and by the reference to a Lord hanging in heaven (lines 37–8). But it may also be looked at from the opposite point of view as a basically Christian charm incorporating pagan elements. In effect, this is what Willy Braekman has done, with no little success in interpreting some hitherto unresolved passages.[47] But first we should establish the names of the nine herbs, as there have been errors perpetrated here by more than one editor.

There is no problem in determining the plants which went into the salve, although it is not possible to assign Linnaean species names to all of them; according to the prose epilogue they are:

mugwort   *Artemisia vulgaris*
plantain   *Plantago maior*

---

[47] Braekman, 'Notes', pp. 461–9.

lamb's cress	*Cardamine hirsuta*
attorlothe	*Fumaria/Corydalis* spp.
chamomile	*Anthemis nobilis* or *Matricaria chamomilla*
nettle	*Urtica* spp. or *Lamium album* (white dead-nettle)
crab apple	*Malus sylvestris*
chervil	*Chaerophyllum temulum*, *C. aureum* or *Myrrhis odorata* in that order of probability
fennel	*Foeniculum vulgare*

The identifications of *mucgwyrt* and *wegbræde* as 'mugwort' and 'plantain' respectively are without doubt; notice that lines 8–11 give an excellent description of the habit and habitat of plantain. Some editors have taken *stune* and *stiðe* to be separate plants, but if, as I indicate above, *stune* is lamb's cress, then again we have a clue to its identity in the words *heo on stane geweox* ('she grows on stone'), and *stiðe heo hatte* ('she is called sturdy'), which adequately describe the plant and its habitat: lamb's cress is a sturdy little plant up to 20 cm tall, growing on 'bare ground, rocks, screes, walls, etc.'[48] In ch. 11 I gave reasons for the identification of *attorlaðe* as a member of the fumitory family. *Mægðe* is a chamomile, but it is not clear which of the plants we now call chamomile may have been meant. *Wergulu* may be a species of the true nettle, or it may be the white dead-nettle (*Lamium album*): both are astringent. The *wudusuræppel* is a 'crab apple'. Two species of chervil (*fille*) grow in England, *C. temulum* is native, *C. aureum* introduced; either may have been meant, and there is a very slight possibility that it may have been sweet cicely (*Myrrhis odorata*), which has a chervil-like odour and taste. Fennel (*finul*) is most probably native, and was a common ingredient of Anglo-Saxon remedies under the name *finul* (*finol*) which, although of Latin origin, appears to have been thoroughly naturalized quite early.

Assuming that the salve to be made from these herbs was intended as an application for haemorrhoids, six of the nine plants (mugwort, plantain, attorlothe, chamomile, nettle or dead-nettle, crab apple) should have had some efficacy in treating them; I know of no properties of lamb's cress, chervil or fennel which would be useful for that ailment. As we saw for *Wið færstice*, this charm also seems to be an addition to an otherwise rational treatment.

From this long charm we learn a couple of things about primitive

48 Clapham, Tutin and Warburg, *Flora of the British Isles*, p. 206.

Anglo-Saxon medicine. The Anglo-Saxons sometimes recited invocations to herbs before using them, and they believed in infection (*onflyge*, 'onfliers'), which passed disease from one person to another. The Christian church forbade the use of heathen rites in the gathering of herbs, but permitted one to invoke the blessing of the Christian God on the gathering.[49] In *Lacnunga* there are two *benedictiones herbarum* which differ from pagan ones only in that they call on the Christian God rather than on a pagan deity.[50] Invocations of herbs in the Latin versions of the *Herbarium* were omitted by its Anglo-Saxon translator. How, then, did the invocations of this charm survive?

Willy Braekman suggests that the charm is of Christian origin but with various pagan elements added to it, such as the section in which Woden is mentioned. He justifies his suggestion by drawing attention to a tradition which persisted into the Middle Ages, that the virtues of certain herbs were connected with an action of Christ shortly before His Ascension.[51] The tradition appears to have been based on the last words of Jesus at that time: 'And these signs shall follow them that believe; In my name shall they cast out devils; they shall speak with new tongues; they shall take up serpents; and if they drink any deadly thing, it shall not hurt them; they shall lay hands on the sick, and they shall recover.'[52] A text of the ninth or tenth century begins: 'Ad uermes occidendos Fervitia (pervinca), dei gratia plena, tu habes triginta quinque indices et triginta quinque medicinas. Quando dominus ad coelos ascendit, memorare, quod dixit . . .' ('To kill worms. O periwinkle, filled with the grace of God, you have thirty-five signs and thirty-five medicines. When the Lord ascended into heaven, remember that he said . . .').[53] The implication is that when Jesus gave his followers power over serpents and poisons (notice that these are the causes of disease in the *Nine Herbs Charm*), he also gave similar powers to certain herbs. And, as Braekman points out, 'the words, *memorare quod dixit* may well be echoed in *gemyne ðu*'.[54] By this interpretation, the *Regenmelde* of the first stanza would then be Christ's 'great proclamation' of the virtues of

49 The Anglo-Saxon laws against magic and witchcraft are conveniently gathered in Grendon, 'Anglo-Saxon Charms', pp. 140–2.

50 Gratton and Singer, *Anglo-Saxon Magic*, p. 202.

51 Braekman, 'Notes', pp. 462–5.

52 Mark XVI.17–18: 'Signa autem eos, qui crediderint, hæc sequentur: In nomine meo dæmonia ejicient; linguis loquentur novis: serpentes tollent; et si mortiferum quid biberint, non eis nocebit; super ægros manus imponent, et bene habebunt.'

53 Braekman, 'Notes', p. 462.   54 *Ibid.*, p. 463.

these herbs. If the charm is originally Christian in concept, then the survival of its invocations to herbs is not surprising.

The periwinkle (*Vinca maior*) also played a role as an amulet in medieval medicine. Ch. clxxix of the Old English *Herbarium* reads:

The herb which is called *priapiscus*, and by another name *vinca pervinca*, is of good benefit for many purposes, that is, first against devil sicknesses and against adders and against wild beasts and against poisons and against every threat and against envy and against terror and that you may have grace; and if you have this herb with you, you will be prosperous and always agreeable; you shall pick this herb saying thus: *Te precor . . . inlesus*. That is then in our language: I pray thee, *vinca pervinca*, who art to be had for many uses, that thou come to me glad, blossoming with thy powers, procure for me that I be shielded and always prosperous and unhurt by poisons and by anger. When you wish to take this herb you shall be clean from every uncleanness, and you shall take it when the moon is nine nights old and eleven nights and thirteen nights and thirty nights and when it is one night old.[55]

The concept of *onflyge* is an interesting one to find in medieval medicine; since it occurs in this charm and elsewhere in Anglo-Saxon medicine, there is no doubt that it refers to a belief that certain diseases were caused by agents which 'roamed through the land' and carried disease from one person to another. There is a salve in *Lacnunga*: *wið fleogendum attre ⁊ færspringum* ('against flying poison and sudden eruption').[56] There is one in bk I of Bald's *Leechbook*: *wið fleogendum atre ⁊ ælcum æternum swile* ('against flying poison and every poisonous swelling'), for which the incantation (which must have been almost pure gibberish to its reciters) is said to be Scottish (i.e. Irish) and in which some Irish words are still recognizable.[57]

[55] *Herbarium*, ed. de Vriend, p. 224: 'Ðeos wyrt þe man priapisci ⁊ oðrum naman uicaperuica nemneð to manegum þingon wel fremað, þæt ys þonne ærest ongean deofolseocnyssa ⁊ wið nædran ⁊ wið wildeor ⁊ wið attru ⁊ wið gehwylce behatu ⁊ wið andan ⁊ wið ogan ⁊ þæt ðu gife hæbbe; ⁊ gif ðu þas wyrte mid þe hafast ðu bist gesælig ⁊ symle gecweme; ðas wyrte þu scealt niman þus cweþende: Te precor uicaperuica multis utilitatibus habenda ut uenias ad me hilaris florens cum tuis uirtutibus, ut ea mihi prestes, ut tutus et felix sim semper a uenenis et ab iracundia inlesus. Þæt ys þonne on ure geþeode, ic bidde þe, uica peruica, manegum nytlicnyssum to hæbenne, þæt ðu me gegearwie þæt ic sy gescyld ⁊ symle gesælig ⁊ ungedered fram attrum ⁊ fram yrsunge. Ðonne ðu þas wyrt niman wylt ðu scealt beon clæne wið æghwylce unclænnysse, ⁊ ðu scealt niman þonne se mona bið nigon nihta eald ⁊ endlyfon nihta ⁊ ðreottyne nyhta ⁊ ðrittig nihta ⁊ ðonne he byð anre nihte eald.'

[56] Grattan and Singer, *Anglo-Saxon Magic*, p. 102.

[57] *Leechdoms*, ed. Cockayne II, 112.

Carmichael reports that the people of the Highlands and Western Isles of Scotland believed that many diseases, such as styes, boils, suppurations and various kinds of swellings, were transmitted by a *grig* ('animalcule', 'mite', 'microbe'); as one Islander explained to him:

> How the hatching-mother of the 'grig' got into the blood and flesh of a person and grew there it was not easy to understand nor easy to explain; but one thing, – where there were ill care and ill keeping the hatching-'grig' was there, running from person to person and from house to house like the wont of the ill tale.[58]

The similarity of this belief to the one implied by *fleogende attre* and the *onflyge* of the *Nine Herbs Charms* is striking. The fact that in the *Leechbook* the incantation against 'flying poison' was said to be Scottish implies that the Anglo-Saxons may have borrowed the idea from the Irish.

That charms have had an even wider distribution in time and space is illustrated by another one from *Lacnunga*:

> For kernels: Nine were node's sisters; then the nine became eight, and the eight seven, and the seven six, and the six five, and the five four, and the four three, and the three two, and the two one, and the one none. May this be a medicine to you for kernel and for scrofula and for worm and for every kind of evil; sing *Benedicite* nine times.[59]

Marcellus gives a very similar charm:

> Conjure swollen glands in the morning, if the day is shortening, if night is, at evening and holding them with the medicinal finger and the thumb say: 'Nine gland sisters, eight gland sisters, . . ., one gland sister; nine glands appear, eight glands appear, . . ., one gland appears, no gland appears.[60]

---

[58] *Carmina*, ed. Carmichael IV, 218.

[59] Grattan and Singer, *Anglo-Saxon Magic*, p. 184: 'Wið cyrnel: Neogone wæran noðþæs sweoster; þa wurdon þa nygone to VIII, 7 þa VIII to VII, 7 þa VII to VI, 7 þa VI to V, 7 þa V to IIII, 7 þa IIII to III, 7 þa III to II, 7 þa II to I, 7 þa I to nanum. Þis þe lib be cyrneles 7 scrofelles 7 worme[s] 7 æghwylces yfeles; sing benedicite nygon siþum.'

[60] *Marcelli De Medicamentis*, ed Niedermann, p. 266: 'Glandulas mane carminabis, si dies minuetur, si nox, ad uesperam et digito medicinali ac pollice continens eas dices: "Nouem glandulae sorores, octo glandulae sorores, septem glandulae sorores, sex glandulae sorores, quinque glandulae sorores, quattuor glandulae sorores, tres glandulae sorores, duae glandulae sorores, una glandula soror; nouem fiunt glandulae, octo fiunt glandulae, septem fiunt glandulae, sex fiunt glandulae, quinque fiunt glandulae, quattuor fiunt glandulae, tres fiunt glandulae, duae fiunt glandulae, una fit glandula, nulla fit glandula."'

In Scotland Carmichael found a very similar incantation for a stye on the eye. 'Why came the one stye without the two styes here? . . . Why came the nine or one at all here?' followed by the *Pater Noster* repeated nine times.[61] In 1956 in Nova Scotia, I saw an application of the same charm when my sister and I were visiting a patient in hospital. My sister complained about the pain of a large stye on her eye, and another visitor, of Highland Scottish origin, suggested she repeat a charm which she had inherited from her mother; it was a close variant of Carmichael's. My sister did, and a few minutes later the stye burst and the pain disappeared. One can understand how such a coincidence of events would have impressed the medieval mind and convinced people of the efficacy of charms. The incident also shows how widespread is the distribution of charms and how difficult it is to say where any particular one may have had its origin.

Two very interesting and difficult charms deserve attention. The first is from *Lacnunga*:[62]

For fever: One shall take seven little wafers such as are offered [at the Mass], and write these names on each wafer: Maximianus, Malchus, Iohannes, Martinianus, Dionisius, Constantinus, Serafion. Then afterwards one shall sing the charm which is named hereafter, first in the left ear, then in the right ear, then over the top of the man's head; and then let a virgin go up to him and hang it on his neck, and let this be done thus for three days. He will soon be better.

> Here came stalking in an (*inspiden*) creature,
> Had his (*haman*) in his hand,

[61] *Carmina*, ed. Carmichael II, 72–3.
[62] Grattan and Singer, *Anglo-Saxon Magic*, pp. 160–2: 'Wið dweorh: Wið dweorh man sceal niman VII lytle oflætan swylce man mid ofrað 7 writtan þas naman on ælcre oflætan: Maximianus, Malchus, Iohannes, Martinianus, Dionisius, Constantinus, Serafion. Þonne eft þæt galdor þæt her æfter cweð man sceal singan ærest on þæt wynstre eare, þænne on þæt swiðre eare, þænne ufan þæs mannes moldan 7 ga þonne an mædenman to 7 ho hit on his sweoran 7 do man swa þry dagas; him bið sona sel.

> Her com ingangan inspiden wiht,
> hæfde him his haman on handa,
> cwæð þæt þu his hæncgest wære.
> Lege þe his teage an sweoran.
> Ongunnan him of þæm lande liþan.
> Sona swa hy of þæm lande coman þa ongunnan him ða liþu acolian.
> Þa com ingangan deores sweostar.
> Þa geændode heo 7 aðas swor
> ðæt næfre þis ðæm adlegan derian ne moste
> ne þæm þe þis galdor begytan mihte
> oððe þe þis galdor ongalan cuþe. Amen, fiað.'

Said that you were his steed.
[I] lay for thee his (*teage*) on the neck.
They began to move from the land.
As soon as they came from the land
Then his limbs began to cool.
Then came stalking in the animal's sister.
Then she made an end and swore oaths
That never this should do harm to the sick one
Nor to the one who might get this charm
Or who knew how to sing this charm. Amen, so be it.

The metrical part of the charm is so corrupt as virtually to defy interpretation, and the emendations of editors have added to the confusion. But some insight can be gained by a careful reading and comparison with other charms. In the first place, the charm is an amulet to be hung about the neck of a person sick of the *dweorh*, so we must first determine what that ailment is. *Dweorh* has almost always been translated as 'dwarf', which may be its primitive meaning, but there is ample evidence in other Old English medical texts that it also means 'fever', apparently fever accompanied by delirium or convulsive seizures. Evidence for this interpretation is found in the very late *Peri Didaxeon*, where the Latin words *interdum et febriunt* ('at times they are feverish') are translated by *hwile he riþaþ swylce he on dueorge sy* ('at times he shakes as if he were feverish'),[63] and in the Old English translation of the *Medicina de quadrupedibus*, where *ad fugandam febrem* ('to get rid of fever') is translated by *dweorg onweg to donne* ('to get rid of *dweorg*').[64] There is also in *Lacnunga* a Christian amulet against *dweorh*, but with no other indication of the ailment. Significant also may be the observation that pennyroyal (OE *dweorgedwostle*) is said to be 'beneficial in cases of spasms, hysteria, flatulence and sickness.'[65]

Elsewhere in Anglo-Saxon manuscripts there are Latin charms against fever in which the Seven Sleepers of Ephesus are invoked as they are in the prose part of this charm. These two differing lines of evidence make it clear that *dweorh* was an Old English word for 'fever', very probably one accompanied by delirium or convulsions. That the metrical part of the charm was also against fever is indicated by the words *þa ongunnan him ða liþu acolian* ('then his limbs began to grow cold'). Whether at some past

---

[63] Löweneck, *Peri Didaxeon*, pp. 30–1.
[64] *Herbarium*, ed. de Vriend, pp. 266 and 337, note to §17.
[65] Grieve, *A Modern Herbal*, p. 626.

time delirious fevers may have been attributed to dwarves we have no way now of knowing.

I have not attempted to translate three words in the metrical charm: *inspiden*, *haman* and *teage*. Cockayne changed *inspiden* to *in spider* without comment and translated the first line by 'Here came entering a spider wight', although the word *spider* is not recorded elsewhere in Old English (the *OED* reference to *spiþra* in its entry on *spider* is to an emendation of manuscript *swiþra*). Grattan changed it to *inwriþen* and translated by 'a creature all swathed'. Most other commentators and editors have accepted Cockayne's spider and have discussed the role of spiders in folk medicine. Audrey Meaney presents important evidence for the role of spider amulets in the control of fever and quotes Dioscorides and Richard Burton in confirmation.[66] In spite of this strong support from other ancient and later sources, it must be emphasized that the presence of the spider as a magic creature in Anglo-Saxon medicine depends on emendation of a most corrupt text. *Haman* elsewhere in Old English means 'covering'; the word *hame*, meaning the collar or part of the collar of a harness, is not recorded before 1300. It is impossible to be sure what it means here; because it seems to have something to do with a steed, it may be 'bridle', as suggested by Grattan. *Teage* has two meanings in Old English, 'cord' or 'bond' and 'box' or 'chest'. Meaney suggests that it may be the case in which the amulet was placed.[67] Anyone interested in unravelling this charm further should read Meaney's excellent analysis of it. Finally, one wonders if *geændode* ('made an end') is an error for *geærnedode* ('interceded', 'brought a message'), which I think might improve the sense; but we do not have enough evidence to justify a change. At any rate, we have here another instance of Christianized magic (the amulet) combined with pagan magic (the charm).

Short metrical charms for child-birth and miscarriage in *Lacnunga* are discussed in ch. 16. In *Lacnunga* there is also a copy, glossed in Old English, of the Latin *Lorica* of Laidcenn,[68] but I am not sure whether this should be called a charm or a prayer.

There is a metrical charm in *Leechbook III* which presents more difficulties of interpretation:

---

[66] Meaney, *Anglo-Saxon Amulets*, pp. 15–17.   [67] *Ibid.*
[68] Grattan and Singer, *Anglo-Saxon Magic*, pp. 130–46. For the latest and most authoritative interpretation of this difficult work, see M. W. Herren, *The Hisperica Famina: II. Related Poems* (Toronto, 1987), pp. 76–89 and 113–37.

If one is in the water elf sickness, then his fingernails are livid and his eyes watering and he wishes to look downward. Do this for him as a treatment: Boarthroat, cassock, the lower part of iris, yewberry, lupin, elecampane, marshmallow heads, fen mint, dill, lily, attorlothe, pennyroyal, horehound, dock, elder, centaury, wormwood, strawberry leaves, comfrey. Pour over with ale, add holy water, sing this charm over three times:

> For wounds I have bound on the best of battle-bandages,
> so that the wounds may not burn nor burst,
> nor expand, nor multiply, nor skip about,
> nor wound grow, nor lesion deepen;
> but to him [I] myself held out a cup of health,
> nor may it pain you more than earth *on eare* would pain.

Sing this many times: 'Earth bear on thee with all her might and main.' This charm may be sung on wounds.[69]

Difficult questions are raised by the charm; what is *wæterælfadl*, and what does the word *eare* mean? It is not clear whether *wæterælfadl* should be read as *wæterælf-adl* ('disease caused by a water-elf') or as *wæter-ælfadl* ('watery elf-disease'). Some commentators have assumed a water-elf corresponding to the nymphs of fountains and streams in Greek and Roman mythology, but there is no mention of them elsewhere except in glosses where the word translates the classical Latin names of these nymphs. On the other hand, the preceding chapter of *Leechbook III* deals at some length with *ælfadl* which, for reasons already given, appears to have designated cutaneous eruptions of various kinds; *wæter-ælfadl* would then be a form of *ælfadl*, a skin ailment having a watery manifestation. Storms suggested chicken-pox, not unreasonably, as it is consistent with the symptoms given, i.e.,

---

[69] *Leechdoms*, ed. Cockayne II, 350–2: 'Gif mon biþ on wæterælfadle þonne beoþ him þa handnæglas wonne 7 þa eagen tearige 7 wile locian niþer. Do him þis to læcedome: eoforþrote, cassuc, fone nioþoweard, eowberge, elehtre, eolone, merscmealwan crop, fenminte, dile, lilie, attorlaþe, polleie, marubie, docce, ellen, fel terre, wermod, streawbergean leaf, consolde. Ofgeot mid ealaþ, do halig wæter to, sing þis gealdor ofer þriwa:

> Ic binne awrat betest beadowræda,
> swa benne ne burnon, ne burston,
> ne fundian, ne feologan, ne hoppetan,
> ne wund waxsian, ne dolh diopian;
> ac him self healde halewæge,
> ne ace þe þon ma þe eorþan on eare ace.

Sing þis manegum siþum: "Eorþe þe onbere eallum hire mihtum 7 mægenum." Þas galdor mon mæg singan on wunde.'

livid nails and sensitivity to light (wishing to look downward).[70] Another possibility is measles, in which also the eyes are very sensitive to light.

The words *wund* and *dolg* are both translated into Modern English by 'wound', but in this charm are differentiated, *ne wund waxsian, ne dolh diopian*. If the *wæterælfadl* is chicken-pox, then the illness starts with a few superficial transparent vesicles which increase in number, then become larger and quite itchy. If they are scratched or otherwise disturbed or infected, they may produce quite deep lesions. According to this analysis, *wund* then stands for a superficial lesion and *dolg* for a deeper, more penetrating one; this meaning for *dolg* (*dolh*) is consistent with its use elsewhere in the Old English medical writings, but this is the only place where the contrast occurs in a single statement.

The word *eare* has been translated as 'grave', and the words *ne ace þe þon ma þe eorþan on eare ace* would then mean 'nor may it pain you more than earth in the grave would pain (you)'. Other possibilities are the survival of *ear* in the meaning 'corn' or 'harvest'; or could it even have the meaning 'harrow'? 'Nor may it pain you more than earth pains in harvest' (or: 'under the harrow'). All three versions make sense of a sort with the general meaning that the illness should not be unduly painful. It is clear that there is much in these Old English charms which we do not understand and which their Anglo-Saxon users may not have understood.

There remains to consider a charm found in a very late version, but of great interest:

> Wen, wen, wen-chicken,
> here you shall not build, nor any dwelling have,
> but you shall go northward to the (*nihgan berhge*),
> where you have, poor wretch, a brother.
> He shall lay for you a leaf at the head.   5
> Under the (*uolmes*) foot, under the eagle's wing,
> under the eagle's claw, ever may you wither.
> May you shrivel as a coal on the hearth,
> may you shrink as dung away,
> and dwindle as water in a pail.   10
> May you become as small as a flax seed,
> and much smaller, as a handworm's hip-bone,
> and may you become so small that you become nothing.[71]

---

[70] Storms, *Anglo-Saxon Magic*, pp. 160–1.

[71] This charm is not in Cockayne's *Leechdoms*; see Grendon, 'Anglo-Saxon Charms', p. 166:
> Wenne, wenne, wenchichenne,
> her ne scealt þu timbrien, ne nenne tun habben,

The main crux in this charm is the word *uolmes* in line 6, which looks like a late form of *folm*, 'palm (of the hand)', 'sole (of the foot)'. Because that meaning makes no obvious sense in the context, it has been emended to *uolues* or *wolues* ('of the wolf'), so that, similarly to the spider in *Wið dweorh*, a wolf has been postulated as a magical animal in Anglo-Saxon medical lore. Audrey Meaney has assembled parallel instances of wolf and eagle magic, so the emendation may be correct.[72] On the other hand, Karl Schneider, disturbed by the break introduced by 'wolf's' in the triad of '*wolues* foot, eagle's wing, eagle's claw', has let the manuscript word stand and suggests that it is a word otherwise unrecorded in Old English meaning *Reisser* ('tearer', 'seizer', 'raptor', 'carnivore'), so that all three references are to the eagle. Schneider also disagrees with the translation of the words *to þan nihgan berhge* as 'to the nearby mountain', and suggests that *nihgan* is a form of another otherwise unrecorded word meaning 'of the killer' or 'of the death-maker', so that line 3 would mean 'but you shall go northward to the hill of the death-maker'.[73] For an understanding of the medical relevance of the charm, this interpretation is of less importance than that of 'wolf' or 'eagle' in line 6. Meaney speculates that the leaf of line 5 may be a scrap of vellum or a leaf from a plant on which the charm was written and that it, together with the foot, wing and claw of lines 6 and 7, may have been an amulet tied to some part of the patient, similarly to the seven sacramental wafers hung around the neck of the person suffering from *dweorh*. One should notice also the diminishing sequence in the second half of the charm, similar to the counting-out sequence in the charm *Wið cyrnel*. Meaney quotes a Babylonian charm which bears remarkable resemblances

> ac þu scealt north eonene to þan nihgan berhge,
> þer þu hauest, ermig, enne broþer.
> He þe sceal legge leaf et heafde.   5
> Under fot uolmes, under ueþer earnes,
> under earnes clea, a þu geweornie.
> Clinge þu alswa col on heorþe,
> scring þu alswa scerne awage,
> and weorne alswa weter on ambre.   10
> Swa litel þu gewurþe alswa linsetcorn,
> and miccli lesse alswa anes handwurmes hupeban,
> and alswa litel þu gewurþe þet þu nawiht gewurþe.

[72] Meaney, *Anglo-Saxon Amulets*, pp. 19–20.

[73] K. Schneider, 'Zu den ae. Zaubersprüchen *Wið Wennum* und *Wið Wæterælfadle*', *Anglia* 87 (1969), 282–302.

to both the charms *Wið wennum* and *Wið cyrnel*, which shows again the universality of Old English charms.[74]

There are about a dozen metrical medical charms in the Old English records; I have dealt with the most interesting and most informative of them in this chapter. Many of the remainder now read as unintelligible gibberish, being apparently from Irish or other foreign languages and written down phonetically as a scribe heard them, but not well enough to be interpreted today, and probably quite unintelligible to those English people who used them. Doubtless this lack of intelligibility contributed no little bit to their supposed efficacy; one should not be able to comprehend magic, lest it cease to be magic.

It is clear that the Anglo-Saxons used purely magical remedies as well as rational ones in medical treatments and that some of these magical ones may have given relief to patients. We must try to put ourselves, however difficult it may be, in the place of the medieval patient. Today the physician imparts confidence in his ability to heal by his white coat, his professional detachment, the atmosphere of his consulting room and the framed diplomas on its walls. These are as much a non-rational part of the healing process as was the intoning of charms. One approach appeals to a society which boasts of its belief in a world governed by 'scientific' cause and effect and which reads its horoscopes in the daily paper; the other appealed to a society where all things were believed to be at the whim of one god or another, beneficent or malignant, who could be propitiated or threatened by the proper ritualistic approaches. The milieux are different and the rituals are different, but the effect is the same – a reassured patient – so presumably the results should be similar. This is a justification for magical treatments in a society which believes in magic as a ruling factor in the operation of the universe, and if it does not work in our society it is because we no longer believe in magic in quite that way.

But the idea still works today. Many illnesses which have very real physiopathic manifestations also have powerful psychopathic components which, if corrected, permit the physician to alleviate or even to remove the other symptoms. In medical practice the patient's (and the attending physician's) attitude to the illness is a critical factor in the success of a treatment. The rigmarole of charms must have supplied this aspect of treatment in medieval times and helped to convince the patient that the forces of nature, the gods themselves, were on his side to help him to

[74] Meaney, *Anglo-Saxon Amulets*, pp. 19–20.

overcome the malignancies of a disease-bearing agent, 'the loathsome one which roams through the land'. Lewis Thomas has described two successful treatments for warts, which are caused by viral infections and are very difficult to eradicate. In one treatment a harmless dye is painted on the wart and the patient assured that it will make the wart disappear. In the other the patient under hypnosis is given similar assurances but no other treatment. Even warts of long standing have succumbed to these treatments. As Thomas wrote:

If it is true, as it seems to be, that the human central nervous system can figure out how . . . to instruct its blood vessels, lymphocytes and heaven knows what other participants in the tissue to eliminate a wart then it is clear that the human nervous system has already evolved a vast distance beyond biomedical science.[75]

If modern medicine is willing to admit the possibility of such cures and even to use them, surely the Old English medical charms deserve a sympathetic appraisal as medicine.

Much has been made of the condemnation of pagan magic by the Church, and its attitude to pagan magic can be assessed from a study of the laws intended to suppress it. But it was not magic *per se* which was forbidden, it was *pagan* magic, as we learn from the *Poenitentiale Ecgberti*: 'Truly it is not permitted for any Christian person that he practice idle divination . . . nor the gathering of herbs with no charm except with the Paternoster and Creed, or with some prayer which belongs to God.'[76] I have referred above to the two 'benedictiones herbarum' and two 'benedictiones unguentum' in *Lacnunga* which differ from pagan ones only in their invocation of the Christian God.[77] Even if the Church did not give wholehearted support to charms and magic practices, it did not condemn them if they refrained from invoking pagan gods and called instead on the Christian God.

[75] L. Thomas, *Late Night Thoughts on Listening to Mahler's Ninth Symphony* (New York, 1983), p. 80.

[76] Grendon, 'Anglo-Saxon Charms', p. 140: 'Nis na soðlice alyfed nanum cristenum men þæt he idele hwatunga bega . . . ne wyrta gaderunge mid nanum galdre, butan mid Paternoster and mid Credan, oððe mid sumon gebede þe to Gode belimpe.'

[77] Grattan and Singer, *Anglo-Saxon Magic*, pp. 202–4.

14

The humours and bloodletting

The remedies quoted in preceding chapters should be sufficient to give a fair idea of most of the methods of Anglo-Saxon medical practice. But there are certain aspects of their medicine which deserve a closer examination, such as phlebotomy, surgery and gynaecological and related conditions. I shall treat these subjects here and in the following chapters, beginning now with phlebotomy.

The practice of bleeding patients was intimately associated with the doctrine of the four humours, although it arose before that doctrine was promulgated in Greek and Roman medicine. It probably had its inception in the belief that the blood carried the factors of disease through the body, and that 'bad blood', blood loaded with these factors, should be removed; this belief was a ruling element of Egyptian practice.[1] The theory of the four humours (bodily fluids) arose out of Hellenic philosophy in an attempt to relate all things to universal laws. Arguments were by analogy, and as there were four seasons, four directions, four winds, four elements and four properties of nature, there were also four humours, so that blood became associated with air and spring which are moist and hot, yellow bile with fire and summer which are hot and dry, black bile with earth and autumn which are dry and cold and phlegm with water and winter which are cold and moist. To this litany of fours were later added the signs of the Zodiac in groups of threes, the four ages of mankind (infancy, adolescence, adulthood and old age) and sometimes, as Christian analogies, the four Evangelists, Matthew, Mark, Luke and John. Most of these analogies were combined into a diagram of the microcosm to accompany a collection of computistical texts compiled by Bryhtferth of Ramsey in the early eleventh century. It is

[1] Majno, *The Healing Hand*, pp. 12–30 and 140.

159

preserved in Oxford, St John's College 17 (7v), and has been reproduced on various occasions, notably by Charles Singer.[2] It is an outstanding example of the extremes to which the Middle Ages could carry analogical reasoning.

The humoral theory was embraced by Galen, and his pre-eminent influence ensured its being enshrined as a basic tenet of medicine for almost another two thousand years; it finally died out in the last half of the nineteenth century.[3] As far as it concerned medicine, the theory was that in the healthy body the four humours – blood, phlegm, red bile and black bile – were in balance, that is to say, the individual was in good humour, had a good temperament, a good mixture of the four humours, but that in disease one or more of the humours was deficient or in excess and the individual was in bad humour or bad temperament. It was the duty of the physician to try to restore health by restoring humoral balance. This might be done by diet and medicines, hence the classification of foods and drugs into hot, cold, moist and dry. But the more expeditious way was to withdraw blood, which was thought to contain the humours, from the affected part or from some other part of the body on which the affected part depended. So for two thousand years perhaps as much blood was spilled in the name of a false theory of health and disease as was lost in the wars fought during the same time.

This humoral theory is not as ridiculous as it may seem at first glance. Blood withdrawn from a normal individual forms a homogeneous clot, but blood withdrawn from one suffering from any number of pathological conditions separates into layers as it clots, the red corpuscles sinking so fast that the clotted blood consists of a lower, red part, and an upper, yellow part. As a modern physiologist has written,

the Greeks related their theory of disease to the fact that the blood separated into layers when obtained from sick patients, the four 'humours' being represented by these separated parts of the blood. The sedimented red cells can be divided into a dark or 'melancholic' humor and a red or 'sanguine' humor, depending on the

[2] Grattan and Singer, *Anglo-Saxon Magic*, pp. 32–3 and fig. 15. It is reproduced also in C. and D. Singer, 'An Unrecognized Anglo-Saxon Medical Text', *Annals of Medical History* 3 (1921), 136–49, where it is accompanied by a valuable analysis and commentary.

[3] *Claudii Galeni Opera Omnia*, ed. Kühn XIX, 485–96: Περὶ Χυμῶν (De humoribus); although this little treatise is most probably not by Galen himself, it contains a good exposition of the Galenic theory of the four humours which occupied so important a place in Western medicine.

degree of oxygenation, while the upper cell-free fibrin clot constituted the phlegmatic and the supernatant serum the choleric humor.[4]

This abnormal clotting is found to occur in cases of injury, in infections, in inflammatory conditions, in rheumatoid arthritis, tuberculosis, pneumonia and in certain normal conditions such as pregnancy, exercise and increased adrenal activity, as well as in some diseases not associated with infection. It is significant that many of the conditions for which bleeding was advocated are those in which this abnormal clotting occurs. It would seem that physicians misread their information, attributing the pathological condition to the abnormal behaviour of the blood rather than attributing the abnormal behaviour to the pathological condition.

The Anglo-Saxons in their medicine paid lip service to the humoral theory but do not seem to have grasped its full implications or to have practised bloodletting as a cure-all. We know it was practised; we have encountered the nun at *Wetandun* suffering from infection in a bloodletting wound (above, p. 27). The clearest statement of bloodletting in the Old English texts is found in Bald's *Leechbook*:[5]

On which season blood(letting) is to be abstained from, on which to be allowed. Bloodletting is to be abstained from for fifty nights before Lammas [1 August] and afterwards for thirty-five nights, because then all harmful things are flying and do much injury to people. Physicians who were the wisest taught that no one in that month should drink a potion nor in any way impair his body, unless he had need for it, and then he should remain indoors at midday, because the air is then most strongly disturbed. For this reason the Romans and all southern people made earth houses for themselves because of the heat and poisonousness of the air. Physicians also say that flowering herbs are then best to work, either for potions or for salves or for powder.

How one should forgo bloodletting on each of the six fives of the month and when it is best. Physicians teach also that no one should let blood when the moon is five nights old and again when it is ten nights and fifteen and twenty and twenty-five and thirty nights old, but between each of the six fives; and there is no bloodletting time so good as in early Lent, when the harmful humours are gathered which were drunk during the winter and best of all on the Kalends of April [1

---

[4] R. G. Macfarlane, 'The Reactions of the Blood to Injury', in *General Pathology*, ed. Sir Howard Florey (Philadelphia, PA, 1962), pp. 216–33. The reader is referred to this article for information on the physiology and pathology of the abnormal clotting reaction and on the conditions and diseases which induce it in the body.

[5] *Leechdoms*, ed. Cockayne II, 146–8; see Appendix 3 (below, p. 195).

April], when trees and herbs first spring up; then the harmful phlegm increases and the harmful blood in the cavities of the body.

If one's blood wound becomes bad, take mallow leaves, boil in water and bathe with it, and pound the lower part, lay on. If you wish to stop blood in a cut, take soot from a kettle, pound to powder, sprinkle on the wound. Take rye meal or barley, burn to powder. If you cannot bind up a blood wound, take a fresh horse dropping, dry in the sun or by the fire, pound to powder very well, lay the powder very thickly on a linen cloth, bind the blood wound with that overnight. If you cannot bind up a gushing vessel, take the same blood that runs out, burn on a hot stone and pound to powder, lay the powder on the vessel and tie up strongly. If during bloodletting a sinew is cut, mix together wax and pitch and sheep's tallow, lay on a cloth and on the wound.

Here we find in essence almost all the rules and problems pertaining to bloodletting. Today it is obvious that the letting of blood could only be harmful in most ailments and that there were times and situations when the harm was likely to be greatest. Apart from the weakening of the body resulting from loss of blood, there was always the danger that the incision would bleed uncontrollably or become infected, as happened with the young nun. Knowing nothing about the necessity for cleanliness to avoid bacterial infection, and probably not even recognizing that some blood vessels were veins with blood flowing at low pressure and others arteries with blood at high pressure, phlebotomists needed to be expert in their trade, and many were not. So there grew up a belief that outside factors influenced the success of bloodletting; and of these factors, two of the most influential were the season and the phases of the moon. In some of this there was a modicum of sense; the hot midsummer weather of June to September in regions around the Mediterranean would be ideal for the spread and growth of bacteria on dirty lancets, phlebotomists' hands and patients' bodies, so that infection then was more likely and the prohibition on bloodletting at that season was a matter of learning from observation.

Bloodletting at the beginning of Lent probably depended on the observation that many people by that time of year were showing signs of scurvy following a winter diet deficient in Vitamin C, but which they attributed, according to what we have just quoted, to harmful humours collected during the winter. After the rigours of Lent there would be even more evidence of dietary deficiencies, requiring further bloodletting to restore humoral balances. The fact that fresh foods are becoming available at the same time (*treow 7 wyrta ærest up spryttað*), and that the eating of these soon disperses the symptoms of Vitamin C deficiency, would lead to the assumption that health was improved by blood being let at the same time. Reasoning *post hoc propter hoc* leads to dangerous conclusions in medicine. Bloodletting may also have been a routine procedure in spring in monasteries, not only to remove the poisons of winter, but to reduce the libidinous tendencies of their members at a trying time of the year.

The supposed influence of the moon must have resulted from more analogical thinking; things must grow more or less according as the moon waxes and wanes, water must rise and fall in living things as the tide rises and falls according to the position of the moon. Even today one finds in agricultural almanacs complicated crop-planting and -harvesting tables arranged by the phases of the moon.

The remainder of the quotation from Bald's *Leechbook* deals with other serious consequences of bloodletting – haemorrhage that cannot be controlled and damage to 'sinews'. I have put the word in quotation marks, because its meaning is ambiguous; *sinew* could mean sinew, tendon or nerve; many nerves run close to blood vessels so that injury to them was easy if an incision was carelessly made. All in all, bloodletting was not a remedy to be carried out casually. The use of dried and powdered fresh horse manure to stanch a bloodletting wound is also given in the third *Leechbook*;[6] it must have been effective. Marcellus recommended soot to stop bleeding piles.

There were other tables predicting the outcome of illness based on the age of the moon and giving days and hours when bloodletting was to be avoided. One such table is as follows:[7]

Old physicians laid it down in Latin books that there are always two days in each month which are especially harmful for drinking any potion or for bloodletting, because there is one hour on each of those days, on which if any vein is opened at that hour, it is loss of life or long illness. A certain physician tested this and bled his horse at that hour and it soon lay dead. Now here are the days as it here says: The first day of March, that is in the month Hlyda, and the fourth day before its end. In the next month, which is called April, the tenth day is harmful and the eleventh before its end. In the month of May the third day is harmful and the seventh before its end. In the month of June the tenth day and the fifteenth before its end. In the month of July the thirteenth day and the tenth before its end. In the month of August the first day and the second before its end. In the month of

---

[6] *Leechdoms*, ed. Cockayne II, 340.

[7] *Ibid.*, III, 152–4; see Appendix 3 (below, pp. 195–6).

September the third day and the tenth before its end. In the month of October the third day and the tenth before its end. In the month of November the fifth day and the third before its end. In the month of December the seventh day and the tenth before its end. In the month of January the first day and the seventh before its end. In the month of February the fourth day and the third before its end . . . One is to be very much cautioned that blood not be let when the moon is four or five nights old, as books tell us, before the moon and the sea are in agreement. Moreover, we have heard it said that no one should live who had his blood let on All Hallows day [1 November], nor if he were wounded. This is no witchcraft, but wise men have found it through the holy wisdom, as God Almighty dictated to them.

Infection was not the only danger in bloodletting. Warnings against drawing too much blood are frequent in the Latin literature, but less so in Old English texts, where one finds only general statements such as these: 'Then in the morning let blood from the arm or from the neck, as much as can be borne',[8] and 'If it is a young man and he has the time and strength blood should be let freely from the arm',[9] and 'Let him blood from the healthy elbow . . . ; if you let too much blood then there is no hope for his life.'[10] The Latin texts are more explicit. For example:[11] 'Open the vein cautiously, so that the patient is not made faint and suffers the danger of health.' But if too much blood was drawn the patient might become unconscious and then something had to be done.

How may we help in swooning? If it is winter time, we bathe the face and soles of the feet with warm water. If it is summer, we bathe the face and soles with cold water, or induce vomiting and apply odours to the nostrils, most suitably pennyroyal, myrtle, sisymbrium [hedge mustard or mint] moistened with vinegar we place around the side.[12]

---

[8] *Leechdoms*, ed. Cockayne II, 130: 'Þonne on morgen forlæt blod of earme oððe of sweoran swa mæst aræfnan mæge.'

[9] *Ibid.*, p. 218: 'Gif þæt biþ geong man 7 þa tid hæfð 7 mihte him mon sceal of earme blod swiþe lætan.'

[10] *Ibid.*, p. 264: 'Læt him blod of þam halan haþoliþan . . . ; gif þu him to fela lætst ne biþ him þonne feores wen.'

[11] CUL, Gg. 5. 35, 426r:'Cum cautela aperies uenam, ita ut non lassetur egrotus, et periculum mortis sustineat.'

[12] Oxford, St John's College 17, 2r. See also Singer, 'A Review', pp. 132–3: 'Quomodo subuenimus in lepotismia (λιποθυμία, 'swoon', 'fainting')? Si hiemis tempore fuerit, calida aqua faciem fouemus uel plantas. Si estate, frigida aqua faciem et plantas fouemus uel uomitum prouocamus et naribus odora opponimus, optimum pulegium, mirtam, sisimbrium, aceto perfusum lateri circumdamus.'

This for a person already ill!

A frequently occurring concept associated with bloodletting in medieval medicine was that of the so-called 'Egyptian days'. More than one version of it is found in the Anglo-Saxon records. The only one in Old English is found in *Lacnunga*:[13]

There are three days in the year that we call Egyptian, that is in our language dangerous days, on which, by no means for no necessity, let neither man's nor beast's blood be diminished; that is, the last Monday in the month we call April, the second is the first Monday of the month we call August, the third is the first Monday after the end of the month of December [the first Monday of January]. Whoever on these three days diminishes his blood, be it man or beast, we have heard say shall soon on the first day or on the fourth end his life; or if his life is longer, that he will not reach the seventh day; or if he drinks any potion on those three days he shall end his life within fifteen days. If anyone is born on these three days, he shall end his life by an evil death, and he who eats goose on these same three days within a space of forty days shall end his life.

As is true for most of these medieval dietary and bloodletting tables, the dates vary from one chart to another, only the first Monday in August being common to all. In various charts of Anglo-Saxon provenance we find instead of the last Monday in April, dates from the end of March to the sixth of April, and instead of the last Monday after the end of December, the last Monday in December.

It was not enough that a patient be bled, he must be bled from the proper vessel. There was a theory that various internal organs were connected with various superficial veins, so that bleeding from these veins drew noxious humours from organs which could not otherwise be reached. The number of bleeding points was about two dozen, varying from one

---

[13] Grattan and Singer, *Anglo-Saxon Magic*, p. 198: 'þry dagas syndon on geare þe we egiptiaci hataŏ, þæt is on ure geþeode plihtlice dagas, on þam natoþæshwon for nanre neode ne mannes ne neates blod sy to wanienne; þæt is þonne utganggendum þam monþe þe we aprelis hataŏ se nyhsta monan dæg an; þonne is oþer ingangendum þam monþe þe we agustus hataŏ se æresta monan dæg; þonne is se þridda se æresta monan dæg æfter utgange þæs monþes decembris. Se þe on þysum þrim dagum his blod gewanige, sy hit man, sy hit nyten, þæs þe we secgan gehyrdan þæt sona on þam formam dæge oþþe þam feorþan dæge his lif geændaŏ; oþþe gif his lif længre biŏ; þæt to þam seofoþan dæge ne becymŏ; oŏŏe gif he hwilcne drænc drincŏ þam þrim dagum his lif he geændaŏ binnan xv dagum. Gif hwa on þis dagum acænned biŏ, yfelum deaŏe he his lif geændaŏ; 7 se þe on þys ylcum þrim dagum gose flæsces onbyriged, binnan feowortiges daga fyrste he his lif geændaŏ.'

account to another. All the surviving bleeding tables from Anglo-Saxon England are in Latin; the one in the *Ramsey Scientific Compendium* is as follows:[14]

From which places should blood be drawn? From twenty-three, to wit from two arteries at the back of the head which we cut for complaints of the head down to the bone four finger-breadths from the ear; similarly(?) two in both temples for watering of the eyes; under the tongue two for rheum of the gums or ailments of the mouth and teeth; one in the middle of the forehead for headache or the madness of frenzy; one in the nostrils for heaviness of the head; two in the neck for abundance of humours in the head or in the eyes or gums; four in the hands, two on the thumb for swelling of the lung, and two others on the little finger for swelling of the spleen and toothache, if the teeth on the right side ache in the left hand, and if the teeth on the left side ache in the right hand in the little finger in the middle joint of the three. For tears two on the nostrils right and left for increases of humours in the eyes; under the ankle-bone of the foot for coldness of the foot itself or for those having kidney complaints or sciatica. So also the woman whose menstrual flow is withdrawn or who does not conceive. On the toes two for injury to the testicles. In the arm we cut three veins, the cephalic, meson and hepatic. We use both the cephalic and hepatic *anacarsis* [ἐγκάρσος, 'obliquely'], that is we make the incision from the side outward, the meson quickly *catatixim* [κατ' ἴξιν, 'in a straight line'], that is without hesitation press the lancet straight down and lift up.

The cephalic, median (meson) and hepatic veins, found in the inner bend of the elbow, were the most important for bloodletting because the cephalic was believed to govern most things to do with the head, the

---

[14] Oxford, St John's College 17, 2r; see also Singer, 'A Review', p. 131: 'Quibus de locis flebotomari debet? De .xx. et tribus, uidelicet de arteriis .ii. in occipiti[o] quos propter querelam capitis incidimus usque ad ossum, mensura .iiii. digitorum de aure; de angelogiis .ii. in ambobus timporibus propter effusionem oculorum; de sub lingua .ii. propter reuma gengiuarum uel uitia oris et dentium; medio de fronte .i. propter dolorem capitis uel alienationem frenesis; de naribus .i. propter grauitatem capitis; de collo .ii. propter abundantium humorum in capite uel in oculis aut gengi[uis]; de manibus .iiii., duas secus digitum pollicem propter inflationem pulmonis, et alias .ii. secus digitum minimum propter inflationem splenum et dolorum dentium, si dentes dextri doluerint in sinstra manu, et si dentes si[nistri] doluerint in dextra manu in minimo digito in [medio] iuncturae trium. De lacrimis .ii. secus nares dextra le[uaque] propter accessiones humorum in oculis; de sub talo pedum propter algorem ipsius pedis uel nefreneticos aut sciaticos. [Si]c mulier cuius menstrua subtraxerit uel non concipit. Super digitos pedum .ii. propter indignationem testium. In brachio incidimus uenas .iii., cefalicam, meson et epaticam. Ce[fa]licam et epaticam anacarsi utimur ad ambas id

median things to do with the lungs and all matters concerning breathing, the hepatic to do with the liver, stomach and other viscera. That is, these three were the principal entry points to humours controlling internal ailments. All in all, to its enthusiasts, phlebotomy was the answer to the maintenance of health and relief from illness for all parts of the body and for all its ills. As one text put it:[15] 'For just as the sky is not always clear nor the sea calm, so our bodies cannot continue in unimpaired prosperity.' The implication, of course, was that bloodletting was the answer.

Although venesection was the accepted method of bloodletting used to restore humoral balance, there were two other methods resorted to for more local withdrawals. Cupping and scarifying could be carried out on any part of the body, but chiefly on the shoulders, abdomen and legs. To draw blood by cupping, the skin was scarified and over these oozing scars there was placed a glass or horn cup, which had been heated so as to rarefy the air within it; as the air cooled suction drew blood from the wounds into the cup. Scarification was much simpler. Cuts were made in the skin over the site from which blood was to be removed and the blood oozing out was wiped away as it emerged, thus slowing formation of a clot. Cupping was useful to withdraw blood from a contusion where there was extravasation of blood, and to draw blood for humoral purposes from regions of the body where there were no suitable vessels near the surface easily reached by venesection, as on the shoulders and abdomen. Scarification had many uses. It seems to have been employed sometimes as a simple counter-irritant, as when the shanks were scarified for paralysis, but it had a more rational use when the area around the bites of animals was scarified to encourage the loss of blood from the wound. In the case of bites by venomous animals, this may have helped to remove venom before it spread through the circulatory system to other parts of the body.

Bleeding seems to have come to the Anglo-Saxons from Mediterranean sources. The number of remedies calling for venesection and cupping in the three *Leechbooks* and the *Lacnunga* are not many. Of over 1,300 remedies in these books, fewer than fifty called for bleeding. There is only one in *Lacnunga*, a drink to be taken an hour before being bled for any reason, and

est a latere in foris flebotomamus, raptim meson catatixim, id est [in]iusso premere flebotomum rectum et sursum leuare' (I have transcribed this quotation directly from the manuscript, 1v).
[15] CUL, Gg. 5. 35, 427r: 'Quia ⟨sicut⟩ nec celum potest esse semper ⟨serenum⟩ nec mare tranquill⟨um⟩, sic corpora nostra in integram prosperitatem perdurare non possunt.'

no mention of cupping or scarifying. In *Leechbook III* one treatment, for paralysis, requires bleeding, but the bleeding is a prophylactic measure to be employed monthly after the episode.[16] It is interesting that these bleedings are to be done on the fifth, fifteenth and twentieth days of the moon, which, as we saw in the quotation above, were days on which bleeding was otherwise forbidden. All other instances of venesection and cupping are in Bald's *Leechbook*, which is the most dependent on Mediterranean practice. Indeed, all remedies requiring these forms of bleeding that I have been able to trace have sources or analogues in Latin texts. The implication is that bleeding was not a native therapy but borrowed from Greek and Roman practices. The situation for scarification is ambiguous, the evidence not being sufficient to say whether it was a native or borrowed practice.

The Anglo-Saxons do not seem to have grasped the theory of the four humours and the development of phlebotomy to remove specific humours in order to restore balance. References to humours in their medicine are more to 'harmful humours' than to specifically unbalanced ones. Therefore, they would have had much less incentive to employ venesection and cupping for the sole purpose of restoring balance and so may have saved many a patient who would have died from loss of blood or from infection if treated by Mediterranean methods.

[16] *Leechdoms*, ed. Cockayne II, 338.

15

Surgery

There are very few references in Anglo-Saxon sources to surgical operations apart from bloodletting. All the remainder deserve some attention.

In Bald's *Leechbook* is the only plastic surgery mentioned in Anglo-Saxon records:[1] 'For harelip: pound mastic very fine, add white of an egg and mix as you do vermilion, cut with a knife, sew securely with silk, then anoint with the salve outside and inside before the silk rot. If it pulls together, arrange it with the hand, anoint again immediately.' This recipe has interesting features. From the description of the procedure, the adjoining surfaces of the two parts of the lip were to be cut so that they might be brought together to fuse as a single piece of tissue. The 'salve' to be applied to the cut edges contains mastic, an antiseptic resin, and the eggwhite would ensure that it would adhere firmly to the surface of the wound. There is some indication that the practitioner was aware of the Hippocratic observation that a sutured wound is likely to open if suppuration takes place, although he may have learned it not from the Hippocratic writings, but from his own observation. Hence the need for a salve which would prevent 'rot'. Notice that if it became necessary to handle the wound (to arrange the edges if they should be pulled awry) the antiseptic salve was to be applied again immediately. No source has yet been found for this recipe; it would be interesting to know if Anglo-Saxon physicians had worked out these minutiae of treatment by themselves.

---

[1] *Leechdoms*, ed. Cockayne II, 56: 'Wið hærscearde: hwit cwudu gecnuwa swiðe smale, do æges þæt hwite to 7 meng swa þu dest teafor, onsnið mid seaxse, seowa mid seolce fæste, smire mid þonne mid þære sealfe utan 7 innan ær se seoloc rotige. Gif tosomne teo rece mid handa, smire eft sona.'

Ch. 35 of bk I of Bald's *Leechbook* deals with ischemia and the treatment of ischemic limbs, and reads:[2]

About blackened and deadened body: The disease comes most often from erysipelas; after the inflammation of the disease has gone away, the body sometimes becomes blackened. Then, from the original inflammation, the disease is to be cooled and treated with cold things, and when the disease comes from outside without obvious symptom, then you must first cool the heat with pounded coriander, with bread crumbs moistened with cold water or with the juice itself of the coriander, or with white of egg or with wine or with other things which have the same properties. When the inflammation and the heat are gone away and the part of the body has turned either somewhat pale or livid or something like that, then scarify the place (then you will improve it), and dry with a poultice such as is made with a cerote and warm barley and such things. He is not to be let blood from a vein but rather shall be tended with purgative potions, either emetic or diuretic, with which you can cleanse the corrupt humour and its red bile sickness. Indeed, even though the harm does not come from the inflammation of erysipelas the sharp potion is good for such patients. If the inflammatory livid or red condition come from outside, from wounds or from cuts or from blows, immediately treat the conditions with scarifying and poultices of barley; according to the way which physicians well know you will amend it. If the livid body is so deadened that there is no feeling in it, then you shall at once cut away all the dead and unfeeling part as far as the living body, so that there be nothing of the dead body left, nor of that which before felt neither iron nor fire. After that let the wound be treated as you would the parts which still may have some feeling and are not altogether dead. With frequent scarifyings, sometimes with many, sometimes with few, wean and draw off the blood from the deadened place. Treat the scarifyings thus: take bean or oat or barley meal, or of such meal that you think that it will accept, add vinegar and honey, cook together and lay on and bind on the sore places. If you should want the salve to be stronger add a little salt, bind on at times and wash with vinegar or with wine. If there is need, give at times a herbal potion and at all times observe when you give the strong medicines what is the power and nature of the body, whether it is strong or hard and easily can stand strong medicines, or is soft and tender and thin and cannot stand the medicines. Apply the medicines according to how you see the bodies, for there is a great difference between man's and woman's and child's bodies and in the constitution of a daily labourer and of the idle, the old and the young, and of one used to suffering and of one unused to such things. Also, pale bodies are softer and weaker than the dark and the red. If you wish to carve or cut off a limb from a body, then observe what sort of place it is and the power of the place, because some places putrefy if one tends them

[2] *Ibid.*, pp. 82–6; see Appendix 4 (below, pp. 197–8).

carelessly, some feel the medicines later, some earlier. If you must carve or cut off a diseased limb from a healthy body, then cut it (not) on the boundary of the healthy body, but much rather cut or carve on the healthy and living body, so that you may cure it better and sooner. When you set fire on a patient, then take tender leek leaves and pounded salt, lay over the places; then the heat of the fire is the sooner drawn away.

I have quoted almost all of this long chapter because it contains much of interest. In ch. 6 its origins and peculiar arrangement were discussed (above, pp. 43–4). A striking omission from all accounts, Latin and English alike, is any reference to how bleeding might have been controlled during the operation. If Celsus had been a source, subsequent operators could have learned from him how to tie off a blood vessel to prevent bleeding and that Roman surgeons had forceps which could be used as haemostats, but there is no evidence that any of this was known to the Anglo-Saxons. Perhaps the cautery was used throughout the operation. Because the chapter is a close translation of a Latin original, we cannot be sure that the operation of amputation as given in the *Leechbook* was ever carried out in Anglo-Saxon England. But the quality of the translation implies that the translator knew what he was dealing with, so that he may have been describing a well-known procedure. (We shall see in a later extract that he was not always able to handle his original so well.) There must have been plenty of opportunity for such a treatment, following not only on erysipelatous inflammation but also on compound fractures, cuts and blows. The instructions are clear and sensible, such as the injunction to amputate in healthy flesh and to pay attention to the condition of the patient. After the cutting and cauterization the wound was treated with an application of tender leek leaves and salt; according to the text, this was to relieve the pain of the cauterization, but the leek leaves would also have an antiseptic action and, according to Dioscorides, would help to emarginate the scab of the burn, leading to better healing with less scar.[3]

A most daring surgical intervention is described in the second part of Bald's *Leechbook*. One of the conditions described there is abscess of the liver and the description of symptoms makes it clear that the abscess was caused by invasion of the liver by *Entamoeba histolytica*, the causative agent of dysentery, which, when it invades the liver, may cause abscesses of great size, particularly in the right lobe, which eventually discharge into the

---

[3] *Dioscuridis de Materia Medica*, ed. Wellmann II, 215.

171

colon, the pleural cavity or the body wall. Surgical treatment of this condition is described thus:[4]

Yet if the swelling and the pus rise so that it seems to you that it can be lanced and let out, then prepare for him first a salve of dove's dung and such like, and beforehand bathe the place with sprinklings with the water and herbs that we wrote about before. When you consider that the swelling is becoming soft and subsiding, then touch him with the iron lancet and cut a little bit and skilfully so that the blood can come out lest a harmful pocket descend in thither. Do not release too much blood at any time, lest the sick man become too exhausted or die, but when you pierce or lance it then have a linen bandage ready so that you may bind up the wound at once, and when you wish to let out more afterwards remove the bandage; let it out thus little by little until it dries up, and when the wound is clean enlarge it so that the opening is not too narrow. Moreover, every day syringe it with a tube and wash with those things; afterwards lay on what may clean the wound. If it discharge very uncleanly, cleanse with honey and draw it together again.

The procedure is not original; it is found in both the *Passionarius*[5] and the *Petrocellus*,[6] and almost certainly had its origin in a Hippocratic operation to remove pus from the pleural cavity.[7] One part of the procedure, about which the sources are quite explicit, is omitted from the Anglo-Saxon account, that is, the insertion of a tent or wick into the wound so that after it had drained a bit, the opening might be closed and a linen bandage applied over it. Each time more matter was withdrawn the wick was removed and replaced. This use of a tent for draining an abscess seems to have been unknown to the Anglo-Saxon translator, who also perhaps did not understand the word *ellychnium* ('lamp-wick') by which it

---

[4] *Leechdoms*, ed. Cockayne II, 208–10: 'Gif þonne se swile 7 þæt worms upstihð to þon þæt þe þince þæt hit mon sniþan mæge 7 ut forlætan, wyrc him þonne sealfe ærest of culfran scearne 7 of þam gelica 7 ær mid spryngum beþe þa stowe mid þy wætre 7 wyrtum þe we ær writon. Þonne þu ongite þæt þæt geswel hnescige 7 swiþrige, þonne hrin ðu him mid þy snid isene 7 snið lyt hwon 7 listum þæt þæt blod mæge ut furþum þylæs þider in yfel pohha gesige. Ne forlæt þu þæs blodes to fela on ænne siþ, þylæs se seoca man to werig weorðe oððe swylte. Ac þonne þu hit tostinge oþþe sniþe þonne hafa þe linenne wætlan gearone þæt þu þæt dolh sona mid forwriðe. 7 þonne þu hit eft ma lætan wille teoh þone wætlan of læt lytlum swa oþþæt hit adrugie, 7 þonne sio wund sie clæne geryme þonne þæt þæt þyrel to nearo ne sie. Ac þu hie ælce dæge mid pipan geond spæt. 7 aþweah mid þam þingum; siþþan oflege þe þa wunde clæsnien. gif hio swiþor unsyfre weorpe clæsna mid hunige 7 gelæt eft togædere.'

[5] *Passionarius* II.61.   [6] *Collectio Salernitana*, ed. De Renzi IV, 250.

[7] *Œuvres complètes d'Hippocrate*, ed. Littré II, 72–4.

was described. And he also did not understand the medicines to be applied to the wound, or else did not have them, because for the Latin 'quotidie ex mulsa lauetur cum sisario, id est superimpones medicamina mollia ut est lemniscosin, basilicon, tetrapharmacum resolutum in oleo roseo donec mundetur',[8] he wrote simply 'every day syringe it with a tube and wash with those things; afterwards lay on what may clean the wound.' It is probable that the compiler had never attempted to carry out the operation and so did not understand some of the directions. It would have been just as well if he had not tried it; the operation continued in use until the nineteenth century, when it was discontinued because it so frequently turned out fatally.

Apart from bloodletting surgery, these are the only surgical treatments found in the Anglo-Saxon medical corpus. Given the lack of antiseptic precautions, of an understanding of the circulation of the blood and of anaesthesia, it is just as well that surgery was rarely employed. Although the details of procedure in Bald's text suggest that amputation was carried out, one wonders how many physicians attempted it and with what measure of success. Indeed, the apparent lack of acquaintance with the finer details of liver surgery leads one to suspect that this operation was a last resort for which the physician was not likely to be well prepared. It is doubtful that Anglo-Saxon practitioners employed major surgery when any other recourse was to be had.

[8] *Passionarius* III.61: 'Every day let it be washed with honey wine, with sisarium, that is put on soothing medicines such as lemniscosin, basilicon, tetrapharmacum dissolved in oil of roses, until it is clean.' Identification of these medicines is still doubtful.

16

Gynaecology and obstetrics

Very often it comes about through the might of God
that a man and woman produce a child in the world.[1]

Not much gynaecological medicine survives from Anglo-Saxon England.[2]
The lost section of Bald's *Leechbook* contained most of that collection's
material on women's complaints. We can appreciate our loss when we read
the table of contents for the missing ch. 60 of bk II:

Medicines for obstruction of women's genitalia and for all infirmities of women: if
a woman cannot bear a child, or if a child become dead in a woman's innards, or if
she cannot bring it forth, put on her girdle these prayers as it is said in these
Leechbooks; and numerous signs how one may know whether it will be a male child
or a female child, and for disease of women, and if a woman cannot urinate, and if a
woman cannot promptly be cleansed [of afterbirth], and for haemorrhage in a
woman, and if a woman is out of her mind, and if you wish a woman to have a child
or a bitch a cub, or if a woman's womb become enlarged, or if a woman suddenly
become silent; forty-one remedies.[3]

---

[1] *ASPR*, ed. Krapp and Dobbie III, 154: 'Ful oft þæt gegongeð mid godes meahtum, þætte
wer ond wif in woruld cennað bearn.'

[2] Much of the material of this chapter is dealt with in detail by M. Deegan, 'Pregnancy and
Childbirth in the Anglo-Saxon Medical Texts: a Preliminary Survey', in *Medicine in Early
Medieval England*, ed. M. Deegan and D. G. Scragg (Manchester, 1987), pp. 17–26.

[3] *Leechdoms*, ed. Cockayne II, 172: 'Læcedomas wiþ wifa gecyndum forsetenum 7 eallum
wifa tydernessum: gif wif bearn ne mæge geberan, oþþe gif bearn weorþe dead on wifes
innoþe, oððe gif hio cennan ne mæge, do on hire gyrdels þas gebedo swa on þisum
læcebocum segþ; 7 manigfeald tacn þæt mon mæge ongitan hwæþer hit hyse cild þe
mæden cild beon wille, 7 wiþ wifa adle, 7 gif wif migan ne mæge, 7 gif wif ne mæge raðe
beon geclænsod, 7 wiþ wifa blodsihtan, 7 gif wif of gemyndum sie, 7 gif þu wille þæt wif

The best we can do to recover something of what has been lost here is to gather from other documents all references to women's diseases and examine them. *Leechbook III* gives most of what remains, apart from some charm material in *Lacnunga*, scattered recipes in the *Herbarium* and some 'fly leaf leechdoms', as Cockayne called them. Ch. 37 of *Leechbook III* deals with problems of pregnancy and child-birth: 'In case a woman cannot bring forth a child, and in case the natural afterbirth will not come away from the woman after the birth and if a dead child be in a woman and in case a woman bleed too much after the birth.'[4] These seem similar enough to the ones lost from Bald's *Leechbook* that we may hope that they repeat some of what was there.

The main text itself reads:

In case a woman cannot bring forth a child, take wild parsnip, the lower part, boil in milk and in water, put equal amounts of both, give the roots to eat and the juice to sup. For the same, bind on the left thigh, up against the genitalia, the lower part of henbane or twelve grains of coriander seed, and that shall be done by a boy or a girl; when the child is delivered remove the herbs lest the innards come out. If the natural afterbirth will not go out of the woman, boil old fat bacon in water, with it foment the vulva; or boil in ale brooklime or mallow leaves, give it to drink hot. If there be a dead child in a woman, boil brooklime and pennyroyal in milk and in water, give to drink twice a day. A pregnant woman is to be earnestly warned that she should eat nothing salty or sweet, nor drink beer, nor eat swine's flesh nor anything fat, nor drink to intoxication, nor travel by road, nor ride too much on horseback, lest the child be born before the proper time. If she bleeds too much after birthing, boil the lower part of *clote* in milk, give to eat, and the juice to sup.[5]

cild hæbbe oþþe tife hwelp, oþþe gif men cwið sie forweaxen, oþþe gif man semninga swigie; an 7 feowertig cræfta.'

[4] *Ibid.*, p. 302: 'Wiþ þam þe wif ne mæge bearn acennan 7 gif of wife nelle gan æfter þam beorþre þæt gecyndelic sie 7 gif of wife sie dead bearn 7 wiþ þam gif wif blede to swiþe æfter þam beorþre.'

[5] *Ibid.*, pp. 328–30: 'Wiþ þon þe wif ne mæge bearn acennan, nim feldmoran nioðowearde, wyl on meolcum 7 on wætre (do begea emfela), sele etan þa moran 7 þæt wos supan. To þon ilcan bind on þæt winstre þeoh up wiþ þæt cennende lim niopowearde beolonan oþþe xii corn cellendran sædes, 7 þæt sceal don cniht oðð mæden; swa þæt bearn sie acenned, do þa wyrta aweg þy læs þæt innelfe utsige. Gif of wife nelle gan æfter þam beorþre þæt gecyndelic sie, seoþe eald spic on wætre, beþe mid þone cwiþ; oðð hleomoc oþþe hocces leaf wyl on ealoþ, sele drincan hit hat. Gif on wife sie dead bearn wyl on meolce 7 on wætre hleomoc 7 polleian, sele drincan on dæg tuwa. Georne is to wyrnanne bearneacnum wife þæt hio aht sealtes ete oðð swetes oþþe beor drince, ne swines flæsc ete ne naht

The first of these remedies has analogues in the *Herbarium*, where we find: 'For women who labour in parturition and are not delivered. Let them foment themselves with the herb wild parsnip and with its water; it will be cured. For purging a woman. The herb wild parsnip, mix with the same water in which it was cooked and give to her to drink, it will purge.'[6] The Old English recipe seems to be a conflation of these two (or perhaps only the second one) with the addition of milk. The second *Leechbook* remedy may be compared with this one from the *Herbarium*:

That a woman may give birth quickly. Let a boy or girl, a virgin, hold against the left thigh near the groin eleven or thirteen grains of coriander seed in a clean cloth tied with a warp thread, and as soon as all the birth will have taken place remove the remedy quickly lest the intestines follow.[7]

Wild carrot and wild parsnip (they were frequently not differentiated) were recommended as emmenagogues and so, probably by analogy, for parturition.

The role of henbane in this treatment may be inferred from another recipe in the *Herbarium*: 'Root of the herb henbane tied to the thigh removes severe pain and swelling.'[8] It is not clear whether the henbane root or coriander seeds were expected to work through analgesic and anodyne properties, or simply as amulets; in any case, the whole procedure of the recipe seems to be magical. Brooklime and pennyroyal are still listed in herbals as emmenagogues, and probably were expected to expel the afterbirth by an analogy similar to that suggested for carrot and parsnip. The warnings to pregnant women concerning diet and activities are eminently sensible, differing little from those given today.

The next chapter deals with problems of menstruation:

fættes, ne druncen gedrince ne on weg ne fere ne on horse to swiðe ride, þy læs bearn of hire sie ær riht tide. Gif hio blede to swiþe æfter þam beorþre nioþowearde clatan wyl on meolce, sele etan 7 supan þæt wos.'

[6] *Herbarium*, ed. de Vriend, p. 123: 'Ad mulieres quae a partu laborant et non purgantur. Herba pastinaca silvatica cocta et de aqua eius se fomentet, sanabitur. Ad purgationem mulieris. Herba pastinaca silvatica cocta, cum eadem aqua ubi cocta est commisce et date ei bibere, purgabitur.'

[7] *Ibid.*, p. 151: 'Mulier ut cito pariat. Herbae coliandri semen grana xi aut xiii in linteolo mundo de tela alligato, puer aut puella virgo ad femur sinsitrum prope inguen teneat, et mox ut omnis partus fuerit peractus, remedium cito solvat, ne intestina sequantur.'

[8] *Ibid.*, p. 51: 'Herbae symfoniacae radix aligata in femore nimium dolorem [et tumorem] tollit.'

In case a woman's menses are suppressed, boil in ale brooklime and the two centauries, give to drink and let the woman bathe in a hot bath and let drink the potion in the bath. Have made up beforehand a poultice of beer dregs and of green mugwort and smallage and of barley meal, mix all together, stir in a pan, plaster on the genitalia and on the lower part of the vulva when she goes from the bath and let drink a cupful of the same draught warm, and wrap the woman up well and let her be plastered thus for a long time of the day; do so two or three times, whichever you find necessary. You should always make a bath for the woman and give the drink at the same times as her menses normally occurred; ask the woman about that. If the woman's monthly flow be too great take a fresh horse dropping, lay on hot coals, let steam strongly between the thighs up under the clothing, so that the patient sweat profusely.[9]

Like brooklime, centaury and smallage are listed as emmenagogues in herbal medicine. Mugwort was the female herb *par excellence*, and was used for all problems of the womb including suppression of menses. Notice the sensible approach to the use of the remedy; the woman is to be treated only at the normal time of the month. What is interesting about the remedies of this chapter is that only the last one (fumigation with steam from horse droppings) does not appear to have analogues in other medical cultures. For the others we can find Latin and Greek recipes which, while not exactly analogous, give insights into the background of these Old English remedies. With the drink to expel afterbirth we may compare a bath given by Cassius Felix to hasten parturition in which, where the Old English recipe has brooklime and marshmallow, the Latin one has fenugreek and marshmallow:

To speed up delivery . . . Fenugreek seed and root of marshmallow which they call althaea, and two handfuls of horehound and linseed; cook all together in water, and that decoction applied in an encathisma, that is a bath, to one seated on a stool

---

[9] *Leechdoms*, ed. Cockayne II, 330–2: 'Wiþ þon þe wifum sie forstanden hira monaþgecynd, wyl on ealað hleomoc 7 twa curmeallan, sele drincan 7 beþe þæt wif on hatum baþe 7 drince þone drenc on þam baþe; hafa þe ær geworht clam of beordræstan 7 of grenre mucgwyrte 7 merce, 7 of berene melwe, meng ealle tosomne, gehrer on pannan, clæm on þæt gecynde lim 7 on þone cwiþ nioþoweardne þonne hio of þam baðe gæþ 7 drince scenc fulne þæs ilcan scences wearmes 7 bewreoh þæt wif wel 7 læt beon swa beclæmed lange tide þæs dæges; do swa tuwa swa þriwa swæþer þu scyle. Þu scealt simle þam wife bæþ wyrcean 7 drenc sellan on þa ilcan tid þe hire sio gecynd æt wære; ahsa þæs æt þam wife. Gif wife to swiþe offlowe sio monaðgecynd, genim niwe horses tord, lege on hate gleda, læt reocan swiþe betweoh þa þeoh up under þæt hrægl þæt se mon swæt swiþe.

177

with the feet open forwards and backwards to the backside, immediately expels what had been held for a long time.[10]

Cassius also has another treatment to provoke menstruation and to eject a dead foetus: 'It takes pennyroyal, marjoram, three scruples of Pontic wormwood tops, nine scruples of soda, honey as needed.'[11]

Here we must digress to examine a problem with plant names. There appears to be a confusion in some Old English texts about the identification of *foenum graecum*. In these remedies where the Old English prescriptions call for brooklime and marshmallow, the Latin and Greek ones call for fenugreek and marshmallow. When first mentioned in Bald's *Leechbook*, it is referred to as 'the herb that is called fenugreek',[12] and subsequently by the same name. But in the *Herbarium*,[13] in the *Peri Didaxeon*[14] and in several glosses[15] it is translated by *wyllecærse* (literally, 'well cress' or 'spring cress', usually rendered in Modern English by 'watercress'); but here in *Leechbook III* we find it equated with *hleomoc*, which is said to be brooklime (*Veronica beccabunga*). Now watercress and brooklime both grow in running water, both have a sharp taste, both have been used as salad herbs and both are said to have the same efficacy in women's disorders. It may be that *wyllecærse* really means 'brooklime' rather than 'watercress', or that the name was used indifferently for both herbs. With the information left to us, I know of no way to settle the identification, but mentioning the problem serves to illustrate the difficulties under which we labour in trying to evaluate Anglo-Saxon medical practice and to unravel the materials in its remedies.

If we take *wyllecærse* to be a translation of (or substitution for) the classical 'fenugreek' we can find other analogues in Greek and Latin texts for the use of it and some of the other herbs mentioned in the *Leechbook* remedies. About fenugreek meal, Dioscorides wrote: 'The decoction of it is

---

[10] *Cassi Felicis De Medicina*, ed. Rose, p. 192: 'Ad accelerandum partum . . . Faeni graeci semen et ibisci radicem quam althaeam vocant et marrubii herbae manipulos II et lini semen simul omnia in aqua decoques, et ipsa decoctio in encathismate, id est in balneo, supra sellam sedenti patefactis pedibus ante et retro podici adhibita confestim excludit qua diu tenebantur.'

[11] *Ibid.*, p. 192: 'Accipit autem pulei, acapni, absinthii pontici cymae Ǝ ternos, nitri Ǝ viiii, mellis quod suffecerit.'

[12] *Leechdoms*, ed. Cockayne II, 180: 'þa wyrt þe hatte fenogrecum'.

[13] *Herbarium*, ed. de Vriend, pp. 86–7.

[14] *Leechdom*, ed. Cockayne III, 134, and *Collectio Salernitana*, ed. De Renzi IV, 222.

[15] Lindheim, 'Das Durhamer Pflanzenglossar', pp. 13 and 50 (§169).

a sitz-bath for the menses, proceeding from inflammation or closure . . . with goose fat it is applied instead of a pessary, softening and opening the places around the womb';[16] about the greater centaury: 'It expels menses and foetuses, shaved in the form of a collyrium and applied to the womb';[17] and about the marshmallow: 'Softened, cooked as they say, with swine or goose fat and turpentine it is made into a pessary for inflammations and closures of the womb, and the decoction of it does the same, expelling also the so-called afterbirth.'[18]

This is not to imply the compiler of *Leechbook III* was familiar with the *Materia medica* of Dioscorides. Much the same information is to be found in Pliny, who recommended as emmenagogues wormwood as a pessary, henbane as a plaster, the lesser centaury as a fomentation or drink or scraped and applied as a pessary to bring away a dead foetus, *daucum* (a group including the wild carrot) as a drink and to bring away the afterbirth, mugwort as a pessary for the uterus and as a drink to expel a dead foetus and in a sitz-bath as an emmenagogue and to hasten the afterbirth or applied with barley meal to the base of the abdomen. He also recommended a decoction of fenugreek, used as a fomentation or in a sitz-bath for women's ailments, especially hardness, swelling and contraction of the uterus.[19] All this leads us to conclude that there is not much in these remedies for women's complaints that is peculiar to northern medicine; they are closely paralleled by Latin and Greek usages, although the herbs used are almost all native to Britain.

Because the *Herbarium* is arranged according to plants and their uses, we cannot expect to find complicated remedies in it, and indeed all of the fifteen which deal with women's complaints are of the same simple form as the two for parturition which have already been quoted. There are a couple for which the Old English translations are incorrect, which, if they were

---

16 *Dioscuridis de Materia Medica*, ed. Wellmann I, 176: τὸ δὲ ἀφέψημα αὐτῆς ἐγκάθισμα εἰς τὰ γυναικεῖα, ὅσα κατὰ φλεγμονὴν ἢ μύσιν συνίσταται . . . σὺν στέατι δὲ χηνείῳ προστίθεται ἀντὶ πεσσοῦ, μαλάσσον καὶ ἀνευρύνον τοὺς περὶ τὴν ὑστέραν τόπους.

17 *Ibid.* II, 11: ἄγει δὲ καὶ ἔμμηνα καὶ ἔμβρυα εἰς σχῆμα κολλυρίου ξυσθεῖσα καὶ προστεθεῖσα τῇ ὑστέρᾳ.

18 *Ibid.*, 155: συμμαλαχθεῖσα δὲ ἐφθή, ὡς εἴρηται, στέατι ὑείῳ ἢ χηνείῳ καὶ τερεβινθίνῃ πρὸς ὑστέρας φλεγμονὰς καὶ μύσεις ἐν προσθέματι ποιεῖ καὶ τὸ ἀφέψημα δὲ αὐτῆς τὰ αὐτὰ ποιεῖ, ἄγον καὶ τὰ καλούμενα λοχεῖα.

19 *Pliny, HN* XXVI.151, XXVII.50 (wormwood), XXVI.152 (henbane), XXVI.153 (lesser centaury), XXVI.157 (daucum), XXVI.159 (mugwort) and XXIV.184 (fenugreek).

ever applied, would not give useful results. One of these in the Latin original is to treat a miscarriage (*abortum*): 'Cook down to a third the root of squirting cucumber and wash oneself below with it.'[20] In the English translation this became: 'If a child is misborn [born prematurely] take the roots of this same herb boiled down to a third, then wash the child with it.'[21] In the English version, it is the child, not the woman, that is to be treated with the medicine. The other mistranslation is of this remedy: 'For the pubes of women. The juice of henbane mixed with saffron; give a dose and you will marvel at the effect.'[22] In the Old English this became: 'If woman's breast be sore, take the juice of this same herb, make into a drink and give to her to drink and anoint the breast with it, then she will soon be well.'[23] The anodyne and sedative properties of henbane would probably work equally well to soothe a patient suffering either from pain in the pudenda or the breasts. With more reason this remedy for sore breasts should be of benefit, as cannabis (hemp) is known to have topical analgesic properties: 'For sore breasts, take the herb wild hemp pounded with fat, put on the breasts, it disperses the swelling.'[24]

I have already given in ch. 13 (above, p. 134) a remedy for suffocation of the womb, which, although it is usually quoted as an amulet, has the authority of Dioscorides of being a rational treatment for hardness and inversion of the womb.

The remaining gynaecological remedies in *Lacnunga* are charms. A series of rites for difficulties with pregnancy and birth are interesting enough to quote in full.

The woman who cannot nourish her child [in the womb]. Go to the grave of a dead person and then step three times over the grave and then say these words three times: 'This be a remedy for me for the loathsome late [slow] birth; this be a remedy for me for the grievous dismal birth; this be a remedy for me for the loathsome imperfect birth.' And when the woman is with child and she goes to her

---

[20] *Herbarium*, ed. de Vriend, p. 159: 'Ad abortum. Herbae cucumeris silvatici, radicem eius ad tertias coquat et inde se sublavet.'

[21] *Ibid.*, p. 158: 'Gif cild misboren sy genim ðysse ylcan wyrte wyrttruman to þriddan dæle gesodenne, þweah ðonne þæt cild þærmid.'

[22] *Ibid.*, p. 51: 'Ad pectinem mulierum. Herbae symfoniacae sucum mixtum cum croco dabis potionem et miraberis effectum.'

[23] *Ibid.*, p. 50: 'Gif wifes breost sare sien genim þære ylcan wyrte seaw, wyrc to drence 7 syle hyre drincan 7 smyre ða breost þærmid, þonne byð hyre sona þe sel.'

[24] *Ibid.*, p. 158: 'Wið þære breosta sare genim þas wyrte cannauen siluaticam gecnucude mid rysle, lege to þam breostan, heo tofereþ þæt geswel.'

husband to bed, then let her say: 'Up I go, over you step; with a living child, not with a dying one; with a full-born one, not with a doomed one.' And when the mother feels that the child is alive, then let her go to church, and when she comes before the altar then let her say: 'To Christ I have said this is proclaimed.'

The woman who cannot nourish her child, let her herself take a bit of her own child's grave, then afterwards wrap in black wool and sell it to traders, and then say: 'I sell it, you buy it, this black wool and seeds of this sorrow.'

The woman who cannot nourish her child. Take then in her hand milk of a cow of a single colour and then sip it with her mouth and then go to running water and spit the milk into it and take up in the same hand a mouthful of the water and swallow it. Then say these words: 'Everywhere have I carried for me the splendid strong kinsman; with this splendid well nourished one. I will have him for me and go home.' When she goes to the brook then let her not look around, nor again when she goes away; and then let her go into another house than that she started from and there let her taste food.[25]

The word *afede*, which I have translated 'nourish', is ambiguous; it may mean either 'feed, support' or 'bring forth, produce'; in the first charm given here I understand that it there means to nurture before birth and have added in parentheses the words 'in the womb'; in the second one, there is no indication whether the nourishing is before or after birth; in the third, because the woman is to take milk into her mouth and spit it into running water, I suppose that the woman is unable to breast-feed her child.

There is one other little charm found on 183r of the *Lacnunga* manuscript. Cockayne transcribed it as written there, but was not satisfied

---

[25] Grattan and Singer, *Anglo-Saxon Magic*, pp. 188–90: 'Se wifman se hire cild afedan ne mæg. Gange to gewitenes mannes birgenne 7 stæppe þonne þriwa ofer þa byrgenne 7 cweðe þonne þriwa þas word: "Þis me to bote þære laþan lætbyrde; þis me to bote þære swæran swærtbyrde; þis me to bote þære laðan lambyrde"; 7 þonne þæt wif seo mid bearne 7 heo to hyre hlaforde on reste ga, þonne cweþe heo: "Up ic gonge, ofer þe stæppe; mid ciwcan cilde, nalæs mid cwellendum; mid fulborenum, nalæs mid fægan." 7 þonne seo modor gefele þæt þæt bearn si cwic, ga þonne to cyrican, 7 þonne heo toforan þan weofode cume cweþe þonne: "Criste ic sæde þis gecyþde."

'Se wifmon se hyre bearn afedan ne mæge, genime heo sylf hyre agenes cildes gebyrgenne dæl, wry æfter þonne on blace wulle 7 bebicge to cepemannum 7 cweþe þonne: "Ic hit bebicge; ge hit bebicgan, þas sweartan wulle 7 þysse sorge corn."

'Se man se ne mæge bearn afedan nime þonne anes bleos cu meoluc on hyre handa 7 gesupe þonne mid hyre muþe 7 gange þonne to yrnendum wætere 7 spiwe þærin þa meolc 7 hlade þonne mid þære ylcan hand þæs wæteres muðfulne 7 forswelge. Cweþe þonne þas word: "Gehwer ferde ic me þone mæran magaþihtan; mid þysse mæran meteþihtan. Þone ic me wille habban 7 ham gan." Þonne heo to þan broce ga, þonne ne beseo heo no, ne eft þonne heo þanan ga; 7 þonne ga heo in oþer hus oþer heo ut ofeode 7 þær gebyrge metes.'

with it: 'I print as I find.'[26] Grattan and Singer dismembered it, giving one part to a charm for an elfshot horse and the rest as a title to the three charms given above.[27] It reads: 'If a woman cannot bear a child: Solve iube deus ter catenas.'[28] G. H. Brown has shown convincingly that the words of the charm are a corruption of 'Solve iubente Deo terrarum Petre catenas' ('Peter, release by God's command the chains of the world').[29] From the point of view of magic, this is a not inappropriate charm for a difficult childbirth. Brown's discussion is important for showing how one should examine all possibilities for interpretation of a manuscript text before attempting major emendations. Grattan and Singer interfered with the *Lacnunga* text in more than one place, with results which are hard to justify. When one is tempted to emend charm texts, one should heed first Brown's words: 'Since we can make sense of the cryptic charm with its affixed title without any displacement or destruction of the heading and text, it seems better to maintain that the Petrine charm is obstetrical.'[30]

The facts that malaria was endemic in much of the English population of medieval times, that people were inadequately nourished and that many food factors such as iron were in short supply must have made the bearing of children difficult for most women. Evidence from grave sites shows that stature was relatively small, that rickets was common, that many women died young, that infant mortality was high. If nothing else, the shortage of iron in the diet must have put women under great stress, particularly during pregnancy, so that miscarriages and premature births must have always been common. In light of these conditions, the charms given here have a poignancy which is striking; the medieval medical practitioner was helpless before the prevailing conditions; only the magician could offer real solace, a solace which was useless, except in so far as it gave some relief to the minds of fearful putative mothers. In a way, charms are an admission of failure on the part of the physicians; in general, they were used for ailments which did not respond to treatment with medicines, and so we can use them as criteria for measuring the relative success of rational medicines.

[26] *Leechdoms*, ed. Cockayne III, 64.

[27] Grattan and Singer, *Anglo-Saxon Magic*, pp. 186–9.

[28] *Leechdoms*, ed. Cockayne III, 64: 'Gif wif ne mæge bearn beran: Solve iube deus ter catenis.'

[29] G. H. Brown, 'Solving the "Solve" Riddle in BL, MS Harley 585', *Viator* 18 (1989), 45–51.

[30] *Ibid.*, p. 50.

The question has been raised why any chapman should buy part of a child's grave. I do not think that the chapman knew what he was buying; the woman most probably concealed the handful of grave mould in a fleece of black wool which she then sold to the trader; the rationale of this procedure seems to be that, as the trader carried away evidence of her previous misfortune, so the misfortune itself would leave her and she should now be able to bear living children.

Of the half-dozen remedies for women's disorders in the *Medicina de quadrupedibus* only a couple need to be discussed. Among the chapters dealing with medicines of animal origin there is one which deals with medicines from the mulberry tree, and among these we find one to treat menstrual flux; the woman is to comb her hair under a mulberry tree with a comb used by no one else and never used again and to hang on an upstanding branch of a mulberry tree the hair caught in the comb; she will then be cured. If she suffers from suppression of menses, she should gather hair in the same way and hang it on a down-hanging branch of the tree.[31] The other unusual remedy is to ensure the birth of a male child: the womb of a hare is to be dried and scraped or rubbed into a potion which both husband and wife are to drink; if the wife alone drinks it then the child will be 'an androgyne, that is as nothing, neither man nor woman' ('androginem, ne byþ þæt to nahte, naþer ne wer ne wit').[32]

In London, BL, Cotton Tiberius A. iii are two short articles on obstetrics and pregnancy. One of them gives criteria for determining the sex of the unborn child, such as if the pregnant woman is offered a choice of a rose or a lily and takes the rose, she is carrying a girl, if she takes the lily, a boy. Another of these indicators survives to our own time: if the womb is carried high she will bear a boy, if low a girl.[33] Finally, there are two items on the effect of the mother's diet on the development of the foetus:

Again there is another thing: if a woman is four or five months pregnant and she then frequently eats nuts or acorns or any fresh fruit then it sometimes happens because of that that the child is stupid. Again there is another thing about this: if she eats bull's flesh or ram's or buck's or boar's or gander's or that of any animal which can beget, then it sometimes happens because of that that the child is humpbacked and deformed(?).[34]

---

[31] *Herbarium*, ed. de Vriend, pp. 239–41. [32] *Ibid.*, pp. 250–1.

[33] *Leechdoms*, ed. Cockayne III, 144.

[34] *Ibid.*: 'Eft oþer wise gif wif biþ bearn eacen feower monoð oþþe fife 7 heo þonne gelome eteð hnyte oþþe æceran oþþe ænige niwe bleda þonne gelimpeð hit hwilum þurh þæt þæt

The second article deals with the formation of the foetus in the womb. According to it the order of development is as follows:[35] the brain is formed first and by the sixth week its membranes are developing; in the second month blood vessels, three hundred and sixty-five of them, large and small, and blood flows through them and the limbs appear; even by the third month the foetus does not have a soul; by the fourth month the limbs are well developed; in the fifth the foetus begins to move and to grow more rapidly and the mother is 'witless', the ribs form and the mother has many afflictions; in the sixth skin and bones are formed; in the seventh the fingers and toes develop; in the eighth the foetus is fully developed with heart and blood; in the ninth the woman knows for certain whether she can bring forth; in the tenth the child must be born or it dies in the womb and the woman does not escape with her life; this happens most often on the eve of Tuesday. I know of no sources for either of these articles.

In the same manuscript there is also a prognostication by the moon's age concerning the character of a child born on each day of the moon.[36] There are many of these charts in medieval documents and many versions of the characteristics for each day. There is no need to pursue the matter further, as it is only another example of the long-held belief in the influence of the phases of the moon on human behaviour.

> þæt cild biþ disig. Eft is oþer wise be þon gef eteð fearres flæsc oððe rammes oþþe buccan oþþe bæres oþþe hanan oþþe ganran oþþe æniges þara neata þe strynan mæg þonne gelimpeð hit hwilum þurh þæt þæt þæt cild bið hoforode 7 healede.'

[35] *Ibid.*, p. 146.   [36] *Ibid.*, pp. 156–8.

17

Conclusions

I hope that I have given enough quotations from their medical texts to allow readers to reach their own conclusions about the quality of Anglo-Saxon medicine. I will, however, present my own for consideration.

We are fortunate to have surviving to our time works representative of three levels of Anglo-Saxon medical literature. At the lowest level is *Lacnunga* which, as medicine, belongs to the least learned type of compilation. It is interesting that we still have this kind of collection with us today; my library contains more than one representative of the type compiled in the twentieth century. But although *Lacnunga* shows no medical expertise in its compilers and only a poor level of competence in either Old English or Latin, it is, for these very reasons, of the greatest value for showing us medical tradition at the level of the untrained and poorly educated practitioner who depended on spells and incantations as much as on potions and poultices for healing. *Lacnunga* gives us a picture of medicine at its lowest level.

Of the Old English works, *Leechbook III* is of special interest because it contains so much Anglo-Saxon medicine relatively uncontaminated by Mediterranean influences. It provides our only opportunity to get a glimpse of Northern European medical practice. It is interesting that, although it deals freely in amulets and charms, it presents on the whole a picture of a medical practice which relied primarily on rational treatments and lets us see that other European cultures than those of Greece and Rome could carry on a rational approach to illness.

The survival of Bald's *Leechbook* is of the greatest importance to our understanding of Anglo-Saxon medicine and it would be of the greatest value to that understanding if we knew that it was a representative of a kind of medicine common to the Anglo-Saxons or that it was unique. At any rate, it refutes the claim that Anglo-Saxon medicine was a degenerate offspring of Greek and Roman medicine, but rather shows that it could take from the Greeks and Romans some of the best they had to offer and integrate that borrowing into an English tradition. Bald's *Leechbook*, particularly the second part, stands equal with such collections as the *Passionarius* and *Petrocellus*, which in the recent past were mistakenly thought to be products of the revival of medicine from the School of Salerno. Its contents also show that Anglo-Saxon physicians were familiar with the standard works in Latin containing the best of Greek and Roman medicine.

Other surviving texts attest to the same conclusion, that the Anglo-Saxons were familiar with Mediterranean practice and appreciated it. Four surviving copies of the *Herbarium*, some of them carefully indexed, show that they were important documents. Collections of short works in Latin on various physiological, pathological and dietetic themes point to the same conclusion that Mediterranean medicine was familiar and appreciated. But there is also the evidence in the whole corpus of Anglo-Saxon medicine that not all aspects of Mediterranean medicine were taken over completely. For example, the theory of humours received less attention than in later times, and bloodletting seems to have been practised with less abandon than in most European medical use.

Many treatments must have given some comfort to patients, and a few were positively useful. But there were conditions, such as cancer, for which no medicines could be expected to be useful and for these resort was had to charms and amulets. That these gave comfort also there can be no doubt, and where they did they no doubt helped patients to heal themselves, or at least, helped them to endure a hopeless condition. Considering how little was known about the physiological behaviour of the human body and that there was no understanding of viral and bacterial infections, of immune reactions and allergies, it is surprising how often a treatment seems to have been designed to take into consideration just these unknown factors. The only explanation I can find is that treatments were in most cases based on careful observations of patients, and evaluation of remedies was done on the basis of those observations. There is no evidence that in general formulas were sterile or applied with no exercise of reasoning.

Never suppose your ancestors to be less intelligent than yourself. There were great men before Agamemnon and we may not look very intelligent to our progeny a millennium hence.

Appendix 1

Quotations for ch. 10

1.1 [Headnote] *Leechdoms*, ed. Cockayne II, 164: 'Læcedomas gif þu wille þæt þin wamb sie simle gesund 7 be coðe 7 sare be wambecoðe 7 innefaran sare 7 to wambe gemetlicunge; syxtyne cræftas.'

1. [Main text] 1. *Leechdoms*, ed. Cockayne II, 226–30: 'Gif þu wille þæt þin wamb sie simle gesund þonne scealt þu hire þus tilian gif þu wilt: Gesceawa ælce dæge þæt þin utgong 7 micge sie gesundlic æfter rihte. Gif sio micge sie lytelu seoð merce 7 finul, wyrc god broð oððe seaw 7 oþra sweta wyrta. Gif se utgang sie læssa nim ða wyrt þe hatte on suþerne terebintina swa micel swa eleberge; sele þonne to reste gan wille. Þas wyrta sindon eac betste to þon 7 eaðbegeatra: bete 7 mealwe 7 brassica 7 þisum gelica gesodene ætgædre mid geonge swines flæsce; þicge þæt broð; 7 eac deah netle gesoden on wætre 7 geselt to þicganne, 7 eac ellenes leaf 7 þæt broð on þa ilcan wisan. Sume alwan leaf sellað þonne mon wile slapan gan, swelc swa bið þreo beana ælce dæge to forswelganne 7 þisum gelice drencas 7 swiðran gif þearf sie syndon to sellane, swiðost on foreweardne lencten ær þon sio yfele wæte se þe on wintra gesomnad bið hie togeote geond oþera lima. Monige men þæs ne gymdon ne ne gymað; þonne becymð of þam yflum wætum oððe sio healfdeade adl oþþe fyllewærc oððe sio hwite riefþo þe mon on suþerne lepra hæt oþðe tetra oþþe heafodhriefðo oþþe oman. Forþon sceal mon ær clæsnian þa yflan wætan aweg ær þon þa yfelan cuman 7 geweaxen on wintra 7 þa limo geond yrnen.

2. Wiþ wambe coþe 7 sare: linsædes gegniden oððe gebeaten bolla ful 7 II scearpes ecedes, oferwylle ætgædere, sele drincan neahtnestigum þam seocan men. Eft: lege dweorge dwostlan gecowene on þone nafolan, sona gestilleþ. Eft: diles sædes lytelne gegnid on wæter, sele drincan. Wiþ wambe coðe 7 wiþ inneforan sare þonne for miclum cele wamb sie ungewealden, do ða þing to þe we be ufan writon. Gif þær þonne sie þæs hrifes wendung oððe gesceorf, genim þreo croppan laures bleda, gegnid, 7 cymenes 7 petersilian syndrige cucleras fulle, 7 pipores XX corna, gegnid eall togædere 7 prie filmenna on bridda wambum adrige, æfter ðon genim wæter, gegnid dile on 7 þas þing gehæte sele drincan oþþæt þæt sar gestilled sie.

3. Wiþ þon ilcan: genim hlaf, geseoð on gate meolce, soppige on suþerne

187

[drenc]. Wiþ wambe coþe seoð rudan on ele 7 þicge on ele. Eft: wilde culfre on ecede 7 on wðtre gesoden sele to þicganne.

4. Wið wambe coðe eft: laures leaf ceowe 7 þæt seaw swelge 7 þa leaf lecge on his nafolan.

5. Eft: heorotes mearh gemylt, sele on hatum wætre drincan. To wambe gemetlicunge: genim betan, adelf 7 ahrise ne þweah þu hie ac swa lange seoð on cetele 7 wylle oþþæt hio sie eal tosoden 7 þicge geurnen; do þonne lytel sealtes to 7 huniges V cuclermæl, eles cuclermæl, sele bollan fulne.

6. Eft: heafdehtes porres gesodenes syndrigne, sele þicgean. Eft: þære readan netlan sæd on hlaf, sele þicgean. Eft: byrigbergena seaw selle drincan. Eft: plum bleda ete neahtnestig. Eft: elnes rinde gebeatene þætte pening gewege on cealdes wætres bollan fullum sele drincan.'

1.2 *Œuvres d'Oribase*, ed. Molinier, *Euporistes* I.16: '*De his quibus expedit ut sanis uenter semper secundus sit. Ab initio igitur antiquorum semper uisum est pro sanitate ut uenter secundus procuretur diebus cotidianis, et inculpabilis urinarum emissio secundum ciborum aut potionum ministrationem redantur.* Quod si haec minime prosequantur, tunc utere est necessarium ea quae haec expellant et procurent uentris et urine obsequia. *Quod si urina minus fuerit ministrata, utantur apozima ubi scandex et apius et fenuculus et sparagus decoquantur; uenter autem si constrictus est, terebintina danda est ad oliue magnitudinem glutiendum dormitum euntibus.* Magis autem educere uolentibus nitrum modicum est admiscendum. *Utilissima autem sunt olera ad deducendum uentrem, qualia sunt beta et malua et brassica semel cocta, porcine uero carnes recentes juscellus.* Quod si haec leuis uisa fuerit et fortiora causa desiderat, ad urina igitur prouocanda addendum est petrosilinum, daucum, anisum, absentium et gramen et politricum et scolimpi radices et citisus et calamentis et origenus; dè unaquaeque earum aut amule inmixtas in aqua discoctas dabis cum uino bibere; purgat enim haec omnis per urinam sanguinem et fit corpori non paruum juuamentum. Ventri autem si quae scripta sunt lenius mouent et amplius secundum habere desiderant, *solutum dabis herba mercuriale in aqua salem coctam et cum comederit ipsam aquam bibat*; sedet sambaci folia similiter facta et accepta hoc modo operatur, nam et polipodoii radicis .lii. puluera et minutatim facta super sardenas et in ptisane sucus coctas si sorbeantur uentrem soluunt. *Aliqui autem et aloen dormito euntibus dant quantum cicaeris tria sunt grana ad glutendum per singulos dies, et habundanter eis redditur uenter secundus. Alii etiam cnicum mittunt in juscello ut simul tritus coquatur.* Omnium igitur predictorum melior est et utilior epitimus in uino potatus. Oportet autem eum qui bibere habet cinare quidem, sed minus quam consuetus est et sic pausare; mouit enim leniter uentrem; quod si mouere amplius uult, jejunus epitumum bibat .liii. in oximelle. *Hoc autem faciat in primum uer antequam ebulescat et effundatur collectus ex hieme humor superhabundans et currat per aliqua membrorum loca et periculosas generant passiones. Multi ergo neglegentes aut*

paralisin aut apoplexia de subito inciderunt in ipsas facta deferunt, et alii pati uidentur
exantematas similia aut aspera, qualia sunt lepre aut impetigines, alii acoras in capite,
aerispilias et aerpitas. Ut ergo hanc predicat aliqua neque aliud nihil malum fiat, purgare
oportet antequam ebullescant collecti humores de hieme resoluentur et currant per membra.'

1.3 *Leechdoms*, ed. Cockayne II, 26–30: (1) 'Læcedomas wiþ eagna miste: gemin
celeþenian seaw oþþe blostman, gemeng wið dorena hunig, gedo on ærenfæt, wlece
listum on wearmum gledum oþþæt hit gesoden sie. Þis bið god læcedom wiþ eagna
dimnesse. (2) Wiþ þon ilcan eft: wildre rudan gedeawre 7 getrifuladre seaw,
gemeng wið aseownes huniges emmicel, smyre mid þa eagan. (3) Wiþ eagna miste:
monige men þy læs hiora eagan þa adle þrowian lociað on ceald wæter 7 þonne
magon fyr geseon; ne wyrt þæt þa seon, ac micel win gedrinc 7 oþre geswette
drincan 7 mettas 7 þa swiþost þa ðe on ðære uferan wambe gewuniað 7 ne magon
meltan ac þær yfele wætan wyrceað 7 þicce. Por 7 cawel 7 eal þa þe syn swa afer sind
to fleoganne 7 þæt þe mon on bedde dæges upweard ne licge 7 cyle 7 wind 7 rec 7
dust; þas þing 7 þisum gelic ælce dæge sceþþað þam eagum. (4) Wiþ eagna miste:
genim grenne finul, gedo on wæter .XXX. nihta on ænne croccan þone þe sie
gepicod utan, gefylle þonne mid renwætere, æfter þon aweorpe of þone finul 7 mid
þy wætere ælce dæge þweah þa eagan 7 ontyne. (5) Eft, of homena æþme 7 stieme 7
of wlætan cymð eagna mist 7 sio scearpnes 7 sogoþa þæt deþ; wiþ þon is þis to
donne: Wið eagna miste, genim celeþonian seawes cuclerfulne, oþerne finoles,
þriddan aprotanian seawes, 7 huniges teares tu cuclermæl, meng togædere, 7
þonne mid feþere gedo in þa eagan on morgenne 7 þonne middæg sie 7 eft on æfen,
æfter þon þonne þæt adrugod sie 7 togoten; for þære sealfe scearpnesse, genim wifes
meoluc þæs þe cild hæbbe, do on þa eagan. (6) Eft, æþele cræft: genim balsami 7
huniges teares emmicel, gemeng togædere 7 smire mid þy. (7) Eft wið þon ilcan:
celeþonian seaw 7 sæwæter, smire mid þa eagan 7 beðe. Biþ þonne selest þæt þu
nime þære celeþonian seaw 7 mucgwyrte 7 rudan ealra emfela, do hunig to 7
baldsamum gif þu hæbbe, gedo on þæt fæt þe þu hit mæg on mid gefoge geseoþan 7
nytta; wel þæt bet. (8) Wiþ eagna miste: gebærned sealt 7 gegniden 7 wiþ dorena
hunig gemenged, smire mid. (9) Eft: finoles 7 rosan 7 rudan seaw 7 doran hunig 7
ticcenes geallan togædere gemenged, smire mid þa eagan. (10) Eft: grene cellendre
gegniden 7 wiþ wifes meoluc gemenged, alege ofer þa eagan. (11) Eft: haran
geallan genime 7 smire mid. (12) Eft: cwice winewinclan gebærnde to ahsan 7 þa
ahsan gemenge wið dorena hunig. (13) Eft: ryslas ealra ea fisca on sunnan gemylte
7 wið hunig gemengde, smire mid. (14) Wið eagna miste eft: betonican seaw
gebeatenne mid hire wyrttruuman 7 awrungenne 7 gearwan seaw 7 celeþonian
emmicel ealra, meng togædere, do on eage. (15) Eft: finoles wyrttruman
gecnuadne, gemeng wið huniges seaw, seoð þonne æt leohtum fyre listelice oþ
huniges þicnesse, gedo þonne on ærene ampullan 7 þonne þearf sie smire mid; þis
todrifþ þa eahmistas þeah þe hie þicce synd. (16) Wiþ eagna miste eft: celeþonian

seaw oþþe þara blostmena, gewring 7 gemeng wið dorena hunig, gedo on æren fæt, wlece þonne listum on wearmum gledum oþþe on ahsan oþ þæt hit gedon sie; þæt bið anspilde lyb wiþ eagena dimnesse. Sume þæs seawes anlipiges nyttiað 7 þa eagan mid þy smiriað. (17) Wiþ eagena miste eft: eorðifies seaw 7 finoles seaw, gedo begea emfela on ampullan, drige þonne on hatre sunnan 7 þa eagan inneweard mid þy smire. (18) Wiþ eagena miste eft: eorðgeallan seaw, þæt is hyrdewyrt, smire on þa eagan, sio syn biþ þy scearpre. Gif þu hunig to dest *þæt* deah. (19) Genim þonne þære ilcan wyrte godne gelm gedo on ceacfulne wines 7 geseoþ ofnete ær þry dagas. 7 þonne hio gesoden sie awring þa wyrt of 7 þæs woses geswettes mid hunige gedrinc ælce dæge neaht nestig bollan fulne.'

Quotations for ch. 13

1.1 *Leechdoms*, ed. Cockayne II, 348–50: 'Gif him biþ ælfsogoþa him beoþ þa eagan geolwe þær hi reade beon sceoldon. Gif þu þone mon lacnian wille þænc his gebæra 7 wite hwilces hades he sie; gif hit biþ wæpned man 7 locað up þonne þu hine ærest sceawast 7 se andwlita biþ geolwe blac, þone mon þu meaht gelacnian æltæwlice gif he ne biþ þær on to lange; gif hit biþ wif 7 locað niþer þonne þu hit ærest sceawast 7 hire andwlita biþ reade wan, þæt þu miht eac gelacnian gif hit bið dægþerne leng on þonne XII monaþ 7 sio onsyn biþ þyslicu þonne meaht þu hine gebetan to hwile 7 ne meaht hwæþere æltæwlice gelacnian. Writ þis gewrit: Scriptum est rex regum et dominus dominantium. byrnice. beronice. luslure. iehe. aius. aius. aius. Sanctus. Sanctus. Sanctus. dominus deus Sabaoth. amen. alleluiah. Sing þis ofer þam drence 7 þam gewrite: Deus omnipotens, pater domini nostri ihesu christi, per inpositionem huius scriptura expelle a famulo tuo N. omnem impetuum castalidum de capite. de capillis. de cerebro. de fronte. de lingua. de sublingua. de guttore. de faucibus. de dentibus. de oculis. de naribus. de auribus. de manibus. de collo. de brachiis. de corde. de anima. de genibus. de coxis. de pedibus. de compaginibus. omnium membrorum intus et foris. amen. Wyrc þonne drenc: fontwæter, rudan, saluian, cassuc, draconzan, þa smeþan wegbrædan niþewearde, feferfugian, diles crop, garleaces .III. clufe, finul, wermod, lufestice, elehtre, ealra emfela, writ .III. crucem mid oleum infirmorum 7 cweð pax tibi. Nim þonne þæt gewrit, writ crucem mid ofer þam drince 7 sing þis þær ofer: Deus omnipotens, pater domini nostri ihesu christi, per inpositionem huius scriptura et per gustum huius expelle diabolum a famulo tuo N., 7 credo 7 pater noster; wæt þæt gewrit on þam drence 7 writ crucem mid him on ælcum lime 7 cweð: signum crucis christi conseruate in uitam eternam, amen. Gif þe ne lyste hat hine selfne oþþe swa gesubne swa he gesibbost hæbbe 7 senige swa he selost cunne. Þes cræft mæg wiþ ælcre feondes costunge.'

1.2 Grattan and Singer, *Anglo-Saxon Magic*, pp. 172–6: 'Wið færstice: feferfuige 7 seo reade netele ðe þurh ærn inwyx 7 wegbræde, wyl in buteran.

Hlude wæron hy, la hlude, ða hy ofer þone hlæw ridan
Wæran anmode ða hy ofer land ridan.
Scyld ðu ðe nu þu ðysne nið genesan mote.   5
Ut lytel spere, gif herinne sie.
Stod under linde under leohtum scylde,
Þær ða mihtigan wif hyra mægen beræddon
7 hy gyllende garas sændan.   .
Ic him oðerne eft wille sændan,   10
Fleogende flane forane togeanes.
Ut lytel spere, gif hit herinne sy.
Sæt smið, sloh seax,
Lytel iserna, wund swiðe
Ut lytel spere, gif herinne sy.   15
Syx smiðas sætan, wælspera worhtan.
Ut spere, næs in spere.
Gif herinne sy isenes dæl,
Hægtessan geweorc, hit sceal gemyltan.
Gif ðu wære on fell scoten, oððe wære on flæsc scoten,   20
Oððe wære on blod scoten,
Oððe wære on lið scoten, næfre ne sy ðin lif atæsed.
Gif hit wære esa gescot, oððe hit wære ylfa gescot,
Oððe hit wære hægtessan gescot, nu ic wille ðin helpan.
Þis ðe to bote esa gescotes, ðis ðe to bote ylfa gescotes,   25
Ðis ðe to bote hægtessan gescotes, ic ðin wylle helpan.
Fled þī on fyrgen hæfde.
Hal wes tu, helpe ðin drihten.

Nim þonne þæt seax, ado in wætan.'

2.3 Grattan and Singer, *Anglo-Saxon Magic*, pp. 150–6:

'Gemyne ðu, mucgwyrt, hwæt þu ameldodest,
hwæt þu renadest æt regenmelde.
Una þu hattest, yldost wyrta,
ðu miht wið III 7 wið XXX,
þu miht wiþ attre 7 wið onflyge,   5
þu miht wiþ þa laþan ðe geond lond færð.
+ Ond þu wegbrade, wyrta modor,
eastan opone, innan mihtigu,
ofer ðy cræte curran, ofer ðy cwene reodan,
ofer ðy bryde bryodedon, ofer þy fearras fnærdon.   10
Eallum þu þon wiðstode 7 wiðstunedest;
swa ðu wiðstonde attre 7 onflyge
7 þæm laðan þe geond lond fereð.
Stune hætte þeos wyrt, heo on stane geweox;

192

stond heo wið attre, stunað heo wærce,   15
stiðe heo hatte, wiðstunað heo attre,
wreceð heo wraðan, weorpeð ut attor.
+ þis is seo wyrt seo wiþ wyrm gefeaht,
þeos mæg wið attre, heo mæg wið onflyge,
heo mæg wið ða laðan ðe geond lond fereþ.   20
Fleoh þu nu attorlaðe, seo læsse ða maran,
seo mare þa læssan, oððæt him beigra bot sy.
Gemyne þu mægðe hwæt þu ameldodest,
hwæt ðu geændadest æt alorforda,
þæt næfre for gefloge feorh ne gesealde   25
syþðan him mon mægðan to mete gegyrede.
þis is seo wyrt ðe wergulu hatte;
ðas onsænde seolh ofer sæs hryge
ondan attres oþres to bote.
ðas VIIII ongan wið nygon attrum.   30
+ Wyrm com snican, toslat he nan.
ða genam Woden VIIII wuldortanas,
sloh ða þa næddran þæt heo on VIIII tofleah.
þær geændade æppel 7 attor
þæt heo næfre ne wolde on hus bugan.   35
+ Fille 7 finule, fela mihtigu twa,
þa wyrte gesceop witig drihten,
halig on heofonum þa he hongode,
sette 7 sænde on VII worulde,
earmum 7 eadigum, eallum to bote.   40
Stond heo wið wærce, stunað heo wið attre,
seo mæg wið III 7 wið XXX,
wið feondes hond 7 wið þæs hond wið freabegde
wið malscrunge minra wihta.
+ Nu magon þas VIIII wyrta wið nygon wuldorgeflogenum,   45
wið VIIII attrum 7 wið nygon onflygnum,
wið ðy readan attre, wið ða runlan attre,
wið ðy hwitan attre, wið ðy wedenan attre,
wið ðy geolwan attre, wið ðy grenan attre,
wið ðy wedenan attre, wið ðy wonnan attre,   50
wið ðy brunan attre, wið ðy basewan attre,
wið wyrmgeblæd, wið wætergeblæd,
wið þorngeblæd, wið þys[tel]geblæd,
wið ysgeblæd, wið attorgeblæd.
gif ænig attor cume eastan fleogan,   55
oððe ænig norðan cume,
oððe ænig westan ofer werðeode,
+ Crist stod ofer alde ængancundes.
Ic ana wat ea rinnende,

7 þa nygon nædran behealdað.   60
Motan ealle weoda nu wyrtum aspringan,
sæs toslupan, eal sealt wæter,
ðonne ic þis attor of ðe geblawe.

Mugcwyrt, wegbrade þe eastan open sy, lombes cyrse, attorlaðan, mageðan, netelan, wudusuræppel. fille 7 finul, ealde sapan, gewyrc ða wyrta to duste, mængc wiþ þa sapan & wiþ þæs æpples gor. Wyrc slypan of wætere 7 of axsan, genim finol, wyl on þære slyppan 7 beþe mid aagemogc þonne he þa sealfe onde ge ær ge æfter. Sing þæt galdor on ælcre þara wyrta, III ær he hy wyrce 7 on þone æppel eal swa, ond singe þon men in þone muð 7 in þa earan buta 7 on ða wunde þæt ilca gealdor ær he þa sealfe onde.'

Quotations for ch. 14

3.1 *Leechdoms*, ed. Cockayne II, 146–8: 'On hwilce tid blod sie to forganne, on hwilce to lætenne. Blodlæs is to forganne fiftyne nihtum ær Hlafmæsse 7 æfter fif 7 þritig nihtum, for þon þonne ealle æterno þing fleogaþ 7 mannum swiðe deriað. Læcas lærdon þa þe wisoste wæron þæt nan man on þam monþe ne drenc ne drunce ne ahwær his lichoman wanige butan his nydþearf wære; 7 þonne on middeldagum inne gewunode for þon þe sio lyft biþ þonne swiþost gemenged. Romane him forþon 7 ealle suð folc worhton eorþ hus for þære lyfte wylme 7 æternesse. Eac secgeað læcas þætte geblowene wyrta þonne sien betste to wyrcenne, ge to drencum ge to sealfum ge to duste.

'Hu mon scule blodlæse on þara six fifa ælcum on monðe forgan 7 hwonne hit betst sie. Læcas lærað eac þæt nan man on þon fif nihta ealdne monan 7 eft .x. nihta 7 fiftyne 7 twentiges 7 fif 7 twentiges 7 þritiges nihta ealdne monan ne læte blod ac betweox þara sex fifa ælcum, 7 nis nan blodlæstid swa god swa on foreweardne lencten þonne þa yfelan wætan beoþ gegaderode þe on wintra gedruncene beoð 7 on Kalendas Aprilis ealra selest, þonne treow 7 wyrta ærest up spryttað; þonne weaxeð sio yfele gillestre 7 þæt yfele blod on þam holcum þæs lichoman.

'Gif monnes blod dolh yfelige genim þonne geormen leaf, awylle on wætre 7 beþe mid, 7 gecnua nioþowearde, lege on. *Gif þu wille on snide blod forlætan, nim ceteles hrum, gegnid to duste, scead on þa wunde. Genim rigen healm eft 7 beren, gebærn to duste. Gif þu ne mæge bloddolh awriþan, genim horses tord niwe, adrige on sunnan oððe be fyre, gegnid to duste swiþe wel, lege þæt dust swiþe þicce on linenne claðe, wriþ mid þy þæt bloddolh neahterne. *Gif þu geotend ædre ne mæge awriþan, genim þæt selfe blod þe ofyrnð, gebærn on hatum stane 7 gegnid to duste, lege on þa ædre þæt dust 7 awrið swiðe. *Gif mon æt blodlætan on sinwe beslea meng tosomne weax 7 pic 7 sceapen smera, lege on clað 7 on þæt dolh.'
(The three recipes I have marked * have each a N[ota] in the margin opposite them in the manuscript.)

3.2 *Leechdoms*, ed. Cockayne III, 152–4: 'Ða ealdan læces gesetton on ledon bocum þæt on ælcum monðe beoð æfre twegen dagas þa syndon swiðe derigendlice ænigne drenc to drincanne oþþe blod to lætenne, for þam þe an tid is on ælcum þara daga gif man ænige æddran geopenað on þara tide þæt hit bið lifleast oððe langum sar. Þæs cunnede sum læce 7 let his horse blod on þære tid 7 hit læg sona dead. Nu syndon hit þas dagas swa swa hit her onsegð: Se forma dæg on Martio, þæt is on Hlydan monðe 7 se feorða dæg ær his ende. On þam oðrum monðe, þe we Aprelis hatað, se teoða dæg is derigendlic 7 se ændlyfte ær his ende. On Maius monðe se þridda dðg is derigendlic 7 se seofoða ær his ende. On Iunius monðe se .x. dæg 7 ær his ende se .xv. On Iulius monðe se .xiii. dæg 7 ær his ende se .x. On Agustus monðe se .i. dæg 7 ær his ende se .x. On September monðe se .iii. dæg 7 ær his ende se .x. On October monðe se .iii. dæg 7 ær his ende se .x. On Nouember monðe se .v. dæg 7 ær his ende se .iii. On December monðe se .vii. dæg 7 ær his ende se .x. On Ianuarius monðe se .i. dæg 7 ær his ende se .vii. On Februarius monðe se .iiii. dæg 7 ær his ende se þridda . . . Is mycclum to warnienne þæt man on .iiii. nihta ealdne monan oþþe on .v. nihta menn blod ne læte, swa us bec seggað, ær þam þe se mona 7 seo sæ beon anræde. Ac we gehydron seggon sumne þisne mann þæt nan mann ne leofode þe him blod læte on ealra halgena mæsse dæg, oþþe gif he gewundod wære. Nis þis nan wiglung, ac wise menn hit afunden þurh þone halgan wisdom swa heom god ælmihtig gedihte.'

Appendix 4

Quotation for ch. 15

Leechdoms, ed. Cockayne II, 82–6: 'Be asweartedum 7 adeadedum lice: Sio adl cymð oftost of omum æfter adle welme on weg gewitenre weorþeð hwilum lic aswertod. Þonne of þam frum welme sio adl mid cealdum þingum biþ to celanne 7 to lacnianne, 7 þonne sio adl cymð utan butan sweotolum tacne, þonne scealt þu ærest þa hæto celan mid cellendre getrifuladre mid hlafes cruman ofþendum mid ceald wætre oþþe mid þy selfan seawe þære cellendre, oþþe mid æges þy hwite oþþe mid wine oþþe mid oþrum þingum þam þe þæt ilce mægen hæbbe. Þonne se [w]elma 7 sio hæto sie aweg gewiten 7 se dæl þæs lichoman sie gewended hwon oððe blæc oþþe won oþþe swilces hwæt, scearfa þonne þa stowe, þonne betst þu ða, 7 drige mid onlegene swa swa mon on weax hlafe 7 of wearmum bere, 7 of swelcum þingum wyrc[ð]. Nis him blod to lætanne on ædre ac ma hira man sceal tilian mid wyrtdrencum utyrnendum oþþe spiwlum oþþe migolum, mid þy þu meaht clænsian þæt omcyn 7 þæs geallancoðe þa readan. Ge, þeah þæt yfel cumen ne sie of þara omena welme swa þeah deah swilcum mannum se secarpa wyrtdrenc. Gif þa omihtan wannan þing oþþe þa readan syn utan cumen of wundum oþþe of sniþingum oððe of slegum sona þu þa þing lacna mid scearpinge 7 onlegena beres; æfter þære wisan þe læces cunnan wel þu hit betst. Gif þæt asweartode lic to þon swiþe adeadige þæt þæs nan gefelnes on ne sie, þonne scealt þu sona eal þæt deade 7 þæt ungefelde of asniþan oþ þæt cwice lic, þæt þær nanuht þæs deadan lices to lafe, ne sie þæs þe ær ne isen ne fyr gefelde. Æfter þon lacnige mon þa dolh swa þu þone dæl þe þonne git hwilce hwega gefelnesse hæbbe 7 eallunga deade ne synd. Þu scealt mid gelomlicre scearpunge hwilum mid miclum, hwilum mid feawum wene 7 teoh þæt blod fram þære adeadedan stowe. Lacna ða scearpan þus: genim bean mela oþþe ætena oððe beres oþþe swilces meluwes swa þe þince þæt hit onniman wille, do eced to 7 hunig, seoþ ætgædere 7 lege on 7 bind on þa saran stowa. Gif þu wolde þæt sio sealf swiðre sie do lytel sealtes to, onbind hwilum 7 þweah mid ecede oþþe mid wine. Gif þearf sie sele hwilum wyrtdrenc 7 gesceawa simle þonne þu þa strangan læcedomas do hwilc þæt mægen sie 7 sio gecynd þæs lichoman, hwæþer hio sie strang þe heard 7 eaþelice mæge þa strangan læcedomas aberan þe hio sie

197

hnesce 7 mearwe 7 þynne 7 ne mæge aberan þa læcedomas. Do þu þa læcedomas swilce þu þa lichoman gesie, for þon ðe micel gedal is on wæpnedes 7 wifes 7 cildes lichoman, 7 on þam mægene þæs dæghwamlican wyrhtan 7 þæs idlan þæs ealdan 7 þæs geongan 7 þæs þe sie gewin þrowungum 7 þæs þe sie ungewuna swelcum þingum. Ge þa hwitan lichoman beoð mearuwran 7 tedran þonne þa blacan 7 þa readan. Gif þu wille lim aceorfan oððe asniðan of lichoman þonne gesceawa þu hwile sio stow sie 7 þære stowe mægen, for þon ðe þara stowa sum raþe rotaþ gif hire mon gimeleaslice tilað, sume lator felað þara læcedoma, sume raþor. Gif þu scyle aceorfan oððe asniþan unhal lim of halum lice þonne [ne] ceorf þu þæt on þam gemære þæs halan lices, ac micle swiþor snið oððe ceorf on þæt hale 7 þæt cwice lic, swa þu hit sel 7 raþor gelacnost. Þonne þu fyr sette on mannan þonne nim þu merwes porres leaf 7 gegniden sealt, ofer lege þa stowe; þonne bið þy þe raþor þæs fyres hæto aweg atogen.'

Bibliography

Alexandri Practica cum optimis declarationibus Jacobi de partibus et Simonis Januensis (Venice, 1522)

Beccaria, A., *I codici de medicina del periodo presalernitano (Secoli IX. X e XI)*, Storia e letteratura, raccolta di studi e testi 53 (Rome, 1956)

Bonser, W., *The Medical Background of Anglo-Saxon England* (London, 1963)

Braekman, W. L., 'Notes on Old English Charms', *Neophilologus* 64 (1980), 461–9

Carmichael, A., ed., *Carmina Gadelica*, 5 vols. (Edinburgh, 1928–54)

Clapham, A. R., T. G. Tutin and E. F. Warburg, *Flora of the British Isles* (Cambridge, 1952)

Claus, E. P. and V. E. Tylor, Jr, *Pharmacognosy* (Philadelphia, PA, 1968)

Cockayne, T. O., ed., *Leechdoms. Wortcunning and Starcraft of Early England*, 3 vols., Rolls Ser. (London, 1864–6)

Colgrave, B. and R. A. B. Mynors, ed., *Bede's Ecclesiastical History of the English People* (Oxford, 1969)

D'Aronco, M. A., 'Inglese antico *galluc*', *Annali. Istituto universitario orientale, filologia germanica* 28–9 (1988), 15–33

De Renzi, S., ed., *Collectio Salernitana*, 5 vols. (Naples, 1856)

Fernie, W. T., *Old Fashioned Herbal Remedies* (Toronto, 1990)

Garmonsway, G. N., *Ælfric's Colloquy* (London, 1939)

Garrod, H. W., ed., *Einhard's Life of Charlemagne* (Oxford, 1925)

Gerard, J., *The Herball or generall Historie of Plantes*, rev. T. Johnson (London, 1633)

Glorie, F., ed., *Collectiones Aenigmatum Merovingicae Aetatis*, 2 vols., CCSL 133–133A (Turnhout, 1968)

Grattan, J. H. G. and C. Singer, *Anglo-Saxon Magic and Medicine Illustrated Specially from the Semi-Pagan Text 'Lacnunga'* (Oxford, 1952)

Grendon, F., 'The Anglo-Saxon Charms', *Journal of American Folk-Lore* 22 (1909), 105–237

Grieve, M., *A Modern Herbal* (Darien, CT, 1970)

Jones, C. W., ed., *Bedae Opera de Temporibus* (Cambridge, MA, 1943)

Jones, W. H. S., ed., *Pliny, Natural History, Books XX–XXXII*, vols. VI–VIII, Loeb Classical Library (Cambridge, MA, 1951–62)

Kühn, C. G., ed., *Claudii Galeni Opera Omnia*, 22 vols. (Leipzig, 1821–33)

Lapidge, M., 'The Hermeneutic Style in Tenth-Century Anglo-Latin Literature', *ASE* 4 (1975), 67–111

Lapidge, M. and J. Rosier, *Aldhelm: the Poetic Works* (Cambridge, 1985)

Lindheim, B. von, 'Das Durhamer Pflanzenglossar Lateinisch und Altenglisch', *Beiträge zur englischen Philologie* 35 (1941), 1–81

Littré, E., ed., *Œuvres complètes d'Hippocrate, traduction nouvelle, avec le texte grec en regard*, 10 vols. (Paris, 1839–61)

Löweneck, M., ed., 'Peri Didaxeon, eine Sammlung von Rezepten in englischer Sprache aus dem 11./12. Jahrhundert. Nach einer Handschrift des Britischen Museums', *Erlanger Beiträge zur Englischen Philologie und vergleichenden Litteraturgeschichte* (Erlangen, 1896), i–vii, 1–57

MacArthur, W., 'A Brief Story of English Malaria', *British Medical Bulletin* 5 (1950), 76–9

Majno, G., *The Healing Hand: Man and Wound in the Ancient World* (Cambridge, MA, 1975)

Mayhoff, K. and L. Jan, ed., *C. Plinii Secundi Naturalis Historiae Libri XXXVII* (Leipzig, 1875–1906)

Meaney, A. L., *Anglo-Saxon Amulets and Curing Stones* (Oxford, 1981)
    'Variant Versions of Old English Medical Remedies and the Compilation of Bald's *Leechbook*', *ASE* 13 (1984), 235–68

Molinier, A., *Œuvres d'Oribase* VI (Paris, 1876)

Mørland, H., *Die lateinischen Oribasiusübersetzungen*, Symbolae Osloenses, Supplement 5 (Oslo, 1932)
    Oribasius Latinus (Erster Teil), Symbolae Osloenses, Supplement 10 (Oslo, 1940)

Niedermann, M., ed., *Marcelli de Medicamentis*, rev. R. Leichtenhan, 2 vols., Corpus Medicorum Latinorum 5 (Berlin, 1968)

Nöth, W., 'Semiotics of the Old English Charm', *Semiotica* 19 (1977), 59–83

Önnersfors, A., ed., *Physica Plinii Bambergensis (Cod. Bamb. med 2, fols. 93ᵛ–232ʳ)* (Hildesheim, 1975)
    ed., *Plinii secundi Iunioris qui feruntur de medicina libri tres*, Corpus Medicorum Latinorum 3 (Berlin, 1964)

Passionarius Galeni . . . in quinque libros . . . una cum febribus tractatu, etc. (Lyon, 1526)

Payne, J. F., *English Medicine in Anglo-Saxon Times* (Oxford, 1904)

Puschmann, T., ed., *Alexander von Tralles, Original-Text und Übersetzung*, 2 vols. (Vienna, 1879)

ed., *Nachträge zu Alexander Trallianus: Fragmente aus Philumenus und Philagrius, etc.*, Berliner Studien 5 (Berlin, 1866)

Rose, V., ed., *Anecdota Graeca et Graeco-Latina*, 2 vols. (Berlin, 1864–70)

Cassii Felicis De Medicina ex Graecis Logicae Sectae Auctoribus Liber Translatus (Leipzig, 1879)

Theodori Prisciani Euporiston Libri III cum Physicorum Fragmento et Additamentis Pseudo-Theodoris, accedunt Vindiciani Afri quas feruntur Reliquiae (Leipzig, 1874)

Schaumann, B. and A. Cameron, 'A Newly-Found Leaf of Old English from Louvain', *Anglia* 95 (1977), 289–312

Sigerist, H. E., ed., 'Das Cambridger Antidotarium', *Studien und Texte zur frühmittelalterlichen Rezeptliteratur*, Studien zur Geschichte des Medizin 13 (Leipzig, 1923)

Singer, C., 'A Review of the Medical Literature of the Dark Ages, with a New Text of about 1110', *Proceedings of the Royal Society of Medicine* 10 (1917), 107–60

Stadler, H., 'Neue Bruchstücke der Quaestiones medicinales des Pseudo-Soranus', *Archiv für lateinische Lexicographie* 14 (1906), 361–8

Storms, G., *Anglo-Saxon Magic* (The Hague, 1948)

Thun, N., 'The Malignant Elves', *Studia Neophilologica* 41 (1969), 378–96

Vriend, H. J. de, ed., *The Old English Herbarium and Medicina de Quadrupedibus*, EETS os 286 (Oxford, 1984)

Wellmann, M., ed., *Pedanii Dioscuridis Anazarbei de Materia Medica Libri V*, 3 vols. (Berlin, 1906–14)

Wright, C. E., ed., with an app. by R. Quirk, *Bald's Leechbook: British Museum Royal Manuscript, 12.D.XVII*, EEMF 5 (Copenhagen, 1955)

Index

acromegaly, 97
ælfadl, meaning of, 97, 142
Ælfric's *Colloquy* 7
ælfsogoþa, diagnosis of, 41; meaning of, 41
ælfþone, attempts to identify, 110; modern and
   Anglo-Saxon uses compared, 110–11
ærn, meaning discussed, 142–3
Æsir, 47
æsmæl, meaning of, 11
æþelferðingwyrt, identification, 112–13
afede, possible meanings of, 181
ἀγελώτος, meaning of, 95
Alcuin, 49
Aldhelm, enigma on hellebore, 111; enigma on
   pepper, 103; *Enigmata*, 25; on wallwort,
   109, student of Theodore and Hadrian, 28
Alexander of Tralles, 23, 67; like and works of,
   69
Alfred the Great, 30; letter from Elias,
   patriarch of Jerusalem, 73
allantoin, physiological behaviour, 128–9
aloe, origin of name, 105
ampulla, used in borrowed OE recipes, 91
amputation, 83; of limbs, 170–1
amulet, against fever, 151; Christian, 133;
   definition, 132; in childbirth, 176
anaesthesia, 12
Anglo-Saxon libraries, 90
Antonius Musa, 60
apple, 145; identified, 147
Apuleius, 66
Apuleius Platonicus, 60
Arabs, 65; drug traders, 105–6
archaeology, 5
artemisia, *see* mugwort, 133

ash sap, for earache, 13
Ashburnham House fire, 32, 89
Asia Minor, 39
asplenium (spleenwort), (*Ceterach officinarum*),
   114, 115
Asser, biographer of Alfred the Great, 73
Assyrian remedy, copper in, 118–19
atramentum, meaning of, 107
Attic honey, 121
atticus, meanings of, 121
attorlape (attorlothe), 145; greater and lesser,
   116; identification discussed, 147; identified
   with *Fumaria/Corydalis*, 112; wrongly
   identified, 112
attrum, meaning of, 107; *see also* atramentum
aucubin, bactericidal glucoside, 123; compared
   with penicillin, 124
augelotus, meaning of, 95
Aurelius, 68, 71

badger, tractate on, 60
Bald, 21, 30, 33; colophon to his *Leechbook*, 20
baldness, 22
Bald's *Leechbook*, 3, 6, 10, 11, 12, 15, 16, 21,
   22, 30, 35, 42–5, 45, 46, 60, 71, 72, 74,
   82, 83, 88, 89, 129; bk I, 77; bk II, 77;
   amulet for malaria, 133; artemisia as amulet,
   133; bk II, compiler's methods, 43–4;
   bloodletting in, 168; bk II, compiler's
   methods, 43–4; colophon to, 20; compared
   with Omont fragment, 91; copper salts for
   infected eyelids, 120; date of compilation,
   73; drugs prescribed in bk I, 100–1; eye
   remedies using copper salts, 120; exotic
   drugs prescribed according to availability,

202

208